Practical Paedodontics

R. H. BIRCH, M.D.S., D.D.O., F.D.S.R.C.S.(E.), F.R.S.H.
Senior Lecturer in Operative Dental Surgery, School of Dental Surgery, Liverpool

D. G. HUGGINS, B.D.S., D.Orth. F.D.S.R.C.S.
*Consultant Orthodontist, Liverpool Dental Hospital.
Liverpool Regional Hospital Board.
Welsh Regional Hospital Board.*

Foreword by

G. E. M. HALLET,
M.D.S., F.D.S.R.C.S., H.D.D., D.Orth. R.C.S.
*Professor and Dean of the Sutherland Dental School
The University of Newcastle-upon-Tyne*

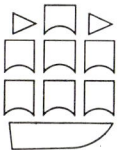

Churchill Livingstone
Edinburgh and London
1973

First Published 1973

ISBN 0 443 00942 2

Printed in Great Britain

Practical Paedodontics

Dedicated to our wives
MARION and MOIRA
with great affection

Foreword

Over the past 25 years, great changes have taken place in the teaching of dental students and nowhere has this been more evident than in the increasing proportion of time and study devoted to the special dental needs of the child and young adult.

Until the last war, dentistry tended to be a profession which treated the end results of disease by operative or mechanistic measures. The conviction that the ideal should be to prevent dental caries and peridontal disease starting in the first place, gathered increasing impetus and a considerable amount of epidemiological research was set in motion to determine the extent of dental problems within the community. Senior academic posts in Children's Dentistry, Child Dental Health, or Preventive Dentistry, have now been established at most schools and also departments devoted to the complete care of the child, not only in relation to his dental and stomatological conditions but also to work in close collaboration with paediatric departments because of the interrelation between many general medical and dental conditions. Child Dental Health (or Paedodontics) whilst embracing the restorative, orthodontic and surgical problems of the young community, must at the same time devote equal emphasis, in so far as it is possible, to their prevention.

The authors of this book have combined to present the subject in a synoptic way confronted by the difficult task of having to decide what especially to emphasise and what to leave out. They are both very experienced and each has specialised in different aspects of Child Dental Health. As one who feels that if dentistry is going to contribute solidly to the general health of the patient at all and that its most forceful impact must be made within the first decade of the individual's life, I am very pleased to welcome this book and wish its authors the success it deserves.

G. E. M. HALLETT

25.7.72

Preface

This essentially practical textbook combines the shared experience of the authors in children's dentistry and orthodontics, and its attitude is one which seeks to remove the traditional barriers between these two fields. It emphasises the importance of regarding the child as a whole individual and not a series of specialist problems. Basic to this concept is the important section on assessment which maintains a central position in the early part of the text, carefully separated from the succeeding chapters on treatment. By these means it is possible for the reader to examine the dental problems in an associated and realistic manner, before referring to the relevant treatment sections.

We wish to express our sincere thanks to Mr Lawrence Finch, Consultant Oral Surgeon, United Liverpool Hospitals, for his valuable contribution to the text and especially for assistance with the sections on oral surgery and dental abscess.

Professor G. E. M. Hallett, Dean of the Sutherland Dental School, Newcastle-upon-Tyne University, has been kind enough to write the foreword for the book and we would like to thank him not only for this but also for his many useful comments and continued interest in the book.

Mr L. J. McBride, Assistant Dental Surgeon at the Chester Royal Infirmary, has helped us enormously with his experienced scrutiny of the text and his criticism of the script content, its quality, and understanding.

Dr. J. M. Mumford, Senior Lecturer and Consultant Dental Surgeon in the Liverpool Dental School, has advised and helped us greatly by evaluating the text during its preparation.

We would like to thank Miss Hilary Cleator, speech therapist to the West Cheshire Hospitals, for her contribution to the section on Speech therapy, and also Mr K. R. Mellor, Chief Dental Technician at the Chester Royal Infirmary, for producing models and appliances used in the illustrations.

Our sincere thanks are due to the publishers, who edited the script and attended to production details with such patience and skill. We are grateful to our many colleagues for their help with useful suggestions and advice, and also to the University of

Liverpool; the United Liverpool Hospitals and Liverpool Regional Hospitals Board for the academic and clinical facilities made available to us.

We wish to thank the photographers, Newcombe and Johnson, Ltd., of Chester, for their help with the illustrations.

Finally we acknowledge with great pleasure the devoted clerical and secretarial work of Mrs N. Carruthers which has contributed so greatly to the production of the book.

RICHARD H. BIRCH
DAVID G. HUGGINS

1973

Introduction

This book has been developed around two central concepts which are, that the patient is a whole individual and not merely the sum of his parts, and that an accurate oral assessment is essential before effective treatment can be carried out. In order to emphasise the latter, the contents have been arranged so that Chapter 2 is concerned with assessment and the relevant treatments are described in the remaining chapters.

Contents

1 The Child in Your Surgery

In an ideal situation the dental surgeon would like to spend a great
deal more of his time seeing his young patients, especially those who
are new to dental health or who already need treatment. It should
be a great time for talking, for making friends and for showing dental
pictures and models. However, the opposite is usually the case and
the child arrives as an emergency with pain after several sleepless
nights. Often he is so afraid because of the tales he has heard from
friends and relatives that he is convinced he is in for an exceedingly
unpleasant experience. This chapter shows how planning ahead with
a sympathy for the child's distress, can do much to reduce the unpleasant aspects of dentistry and also to develop trust between the
dental surgeon and his reluctant young patient.

Age and Treatment Acceptance

It is recognised that there is a series of changing horizons through
which the child's mental and emotional status develops, the early
environment being almost completely maternal. This complete
dependence upon the mother until the age of three years makes it
necessary to consider mother and child as a single unit.

By approximately four years of age the child will have increased
his independence to the extent that he will begin to test authority
by resisting it. This is called the 'resistant phase' and is part of
normal development although not all children show it outwardly.
It does not usually last more than one year, but unsympathetic
attempts to treat the child will increase his resistance and sense of
frustration so that he will become difficult to manage. Open conflict with the child should be avoided since it is an indication that
the dentist has lost control of the situation and the confidence of
parent and child will evaporate. When the observant practitioner
notes signs of mounting resistance he should take steps to deflate the
situation by a temporary change of emphasis in the treatment.
Greater stress should be laid on oral hygiene and diet and on the
practical steps both the parent and child can take to improve the
oral environment. Operative technique in the surgery can be reduced
to minimal preparation but should not be completely abandoned
during this phase.

An increase in age brings an improvement in cooperation. However, it is not uncommon to find that a sudden alteration in willingness to accept treatment may reflect an emotional crisis at home at or school. Under these circumstances treatment should not be abandoned but confined to pleasant procedures, e.g. scaling and polishing providing that dental health is not prejudiced.

Sometimes the young patient reacts differently in the surgery depending on whether the father or mother is present. Resistance to treatment may increase considerably if the child thinks he can gain the sympathy of the parents and in these circumstances it may be better to exclude them from the chairside whilst operative techniques are being carried out. Before discussing the child's problems with the parent, the dentist should always take the precaution of finding out the marital status of the mother, e.g. whether divorced or whether the child is being fostered.

Whatever the age of the child, the communication of fear from parents and other children can prejudice treatment long before the child arrives at the surgery. Parental misconceptions and failures in their own dental health may communicate a very real sense of uncertainty and fear to the young patient, but confidence can only be restored by discussion and planning. It should never be taken for granted that the parent and child understand the dental problem, its solution or its consequences, but they should be asked to discuss anxieties and uncertainties so that the child may be helped with appreciation and sympathy from all sides.

Staff and Surgery Arrangements

Surgeries are built and equipped so much according to personal preference that only general comments can be offered as to the arrangement of these premises. The minimum surgery staff requirements are one nurse whose duties are almost wholly chairside and a second nurse who is concerned with reception, appointments, telephone and filing. If the arrangements serve a group practice one receptionist can effectively serve four busy surgeries from a centrally placed office area, and an oral hygienist can undertake the prophylaxis and oral hygiene instruction for several dental surgeons in a suite of surgeries. In addition to this she is easily trained to carry out routine radiographic and developing procedures.

Good staff are worth their weight in gold. If, however, they are inefficient, the fault lies either in their selection or training. Newly appointed personnel should not be allowed to drift through a practice training scheme which consists merely of picking up the routine as they go along. A conscientious effort should be made to give them a specific training programme designed not only to cover surgery techniques and needs but also to provide a real understanding of practice management. Unless the practice staff are involved in the aims as well as the problems of the surgery their functional efficiency will not rise to its potential level. Before training schemes are designed, the dental surgeon should carry out an individual work analysis for each person in the surgery. This comprehensive assessment should include areas of work and movement, use of sinks (two are needed), the stocking of supplies and equipment, their handling and proper cleansing. Although an attitude of flexibility is greatly to be encouraged, the operator must be certain that all peripheral systems are subservient to the chairside programme and, for example, that telephones are not allowed to interfere with treatment. Training staff to respect these concepts is time well spent, but by the same token the dentist should keep a critical eye on his own activities so that he can give clear directions which will not cause duplication of his or other staff activities. He should be prepared to discuss the working arrangements with his staff and listen sympathetically and constructively if they find that any situation is difficult to control.

The sight and sounds of instruments within the surgery frightens children and for this reason the armamentarium should not be on display especially when a new patient is being introduced. Sudden, hurried movements of the staff behind the chair are associated in the apprehensive child's mind with impending urgent activity in his mouth and he is constantly turning his head in a fearful anticipation. Where possible, therefore, a calm, quiet atmosphere should be maintained and no background conversation allowed, other than that required and directed by the operator. The chairside nurse must anticipate the needs of the next patient so that there is no delay in arranging fresh instruments as the treated child is leaving the surgery.

The health of the operator and staff are important and proper attention should be given to providing congenial working conditions which must include resting facilities and refreshments, besides the more obvious factors such as ventilation, heating and floor surfaces. In this respect operating positions are of particular importance to the dental surgeon for whom poor postural habits can form severe disabilities and limit his clinical efficiency. He must satisfy himself that his equipment is arranged to serve him effectively, without inducing postural stress. Great care should be taken to ensure that

waste mercury and amalgam are collected in water-filled con-
tainers in order to reduce atmospheric mercury vaporisation. A
positive ventilation system should be installed and pleasant air mists
used to get rid of traditional surgery smells. Subdued background
music has an advantage over an almost silent atmosphere in the
surgery suite, because instrument and other sounds are less noticeable.

The waiting-room requires a comfortable and friendly atmosphere
with magazines, comics and fish tanks for patients to look at, and
since it is an area where considerable movement occurs, consideration
should be given to such factors as doors and floor covering.

It is important when considering the child's treatment that the
parents should be made aware of the role that they can play in this
programme. Such an approach is even more essential where
children are physically or mentally handicapped, for here dental
neglect can lead to serious health risks, as in cases with rheumatic
heart disease. The planning, management and recall systems should
be operated in such a way that those children with serious medical
conditions should be under close surveillance and emergency treatment readily available if needed.

Routine appointments may be made for up to six months, but for
longer periods the patient is liable to forget unless a reminder is sent.
A practical way of carrying this out is to file an appointment card
bearing the patient's name and address in a monthly index, the
exact date being added prior to posting. Planning begins with the
appointments system which is the first line of communication
between the dentist and the patient. As such, details of availability,
alternative telephone numbers must be readily at hand in case
appointment changes are required at short notice. Patients should
not be allowed to alter their agreed dates except under exceptional
circumstances such as illness. If alterations are made it is imperative
that adequate consultation is made between all members of the
surgery staff before the arrangements are confirmed. It is bad
practice to 'fit patients in' between other established appointments.

The patient's chart should be the pivot of the practice planning
so that, besides name, address and clinical data, it should show
clearly the following against each appointment:

Date
Details of clinical work
Memos for next appointment: check radiographs, dentures, study
    models, amalgams, or extractions under L.A.
Date of next appointment and duration.
Personal memoranda.

These observations written before the patient leaves, are for the use of surgery staff so that exact equipment requirements will be known for the next visit and the patient told if special precautions will be necessary on that day. The basic system may work well but is rapidly brought to a halt by the arrival of two or three unscheduled cases complaining of pain and requiring emergency treatment. By setting aside a specific time for such cases each day correlated with the possible use of an anaesthetist they will not delay the treatment of routine patients.

The surgery office acts as the administrative centre for the practice. Information required for the case assessment or for the follow-up of treated cases should be contained in alphabetically filed case sheets, with radiographs and photographs, all appropriately cross-indexed. Study models are kept in cardboard boxes in series of four, each separated to prevent damage. They are stored numerically to allow easy addition to the system and quick cross-reference. Transparencies, both full face and profile, should be kept in plastic hangers together with photographs of appliances where this is appropriate. Stock lists should be mounted on cards for effective handling and correspondence filed alphabetically together with copies of all letters sent from the surgery. These may require cross-reference to a cash book where details of purchases are recorded.

First Visits

The young child's first visit to the dentist or doctor may represent his introduction to the world outside his domestic environment. Whether he is brought to the surgery as an emergency case or as part of a thoughtfully planned invitation, will depend largely on the attitude of the parents.

In emergency cases, the young patient is often fretful because of lack of sleep due to pain or fear and may be difficult to control. In these circumstances an adequate dental examination may only be possible if the child can be placed horizontally with his back on the seated parent's knees. In this position the parent is able to control arms and legs leaving the operator, who is seated alongside, with both his hands free to make the oral examination.

If extractions are necessary to relieve the pain then the procedure may be straightforward once the relevant medical and dental histories have been obtained. Where general anaesthesia is the method of choice, it is reasonable to extract other grossly carious teeth at the same time unless they exceed five, when a further appointment should be considered for completing this work. However, each case must be assessed individually to determine the degree of discomfort that the patient is likely to suffer from multiple extractions. Where the patient has orthodontic or other dental problems requiring extractions apart from those immediately related to the pain, then these should be delayed for detailed assessment at a later date.

The first visit should be made on the basis that it is introductory and for inspection only and this should be stated on the appointment card. Its purpose will be to collect information and establish relationships with child and parent. Diagnosis and treatment plan are usually provisional at this stage and can be completed later when details from further investigations have been obtained.

Details of diet especially biscuit, sweet consumption, and eating habits, should be obtained from the child where possible and completed later by consulting the parent but, in questioning the adult, the dentist should avoid implied criticism at this stage since it may provoke a hostile attitude in which the parent will assume a protective role towards the child. Under these circumstances she may unconsciously play down an important factor such as biscuit consumption for fear of embarrassment when the problem is discussed.

Introduction to Treatment

Consideration should be given to the following points:

1. The child should be seen punctually, preferably in the early part of day if very young.
2. Discussion with parent to establish harmonious relationship and to explain concepts of treatment.
3. Short chairside sessions perhaps limited to ten minutes on first occasion unless emergency treatment is required.
4. The dental surgeon must keep faith with his patient and not promise painless episodes which he cannot guarantee.
5. The parent should be tactfully persuaded to return to the waiting room as early in the treatment as possible, except where the patient is very young. She should be encouraged not to interrupt the establishment of the dentist/patient relationship by talking to her child even though she is offering well-intentioned encouragement.
6. The maintenence of a calm but cheerful manner towards young children is a great help especially with difficult management problems. Loss of temper is to be avoided at all costs as this leads to open conflict with the child and loss of confidence.

As the time for operative procedures arrives, the opportunity should always be taken to explain to the young patient exactly what the treatment involves, but such emotive words as 'pain', 'hurt', 'needle', 'cry', and 'injection', should be avoided and replaced by 'rub', 'tingle', and 'stroke'. Active participation by holding mirror and cotton rolls can also help to remove some of the child's feeling of remoteness and isolation in his new environment. As a preliminary to an initial scaling and polishing the patient should be shown the sensation of the rubber cup polishing the finger nail. Even though the programme for a small child is very restricted during the early visits, the operator should have a precise schedule in mind so that each visit will show a slight but significant advance over the patient's previous experience. It may be an advantage, especially with the uncooperative child, to indicate upon his chart the intended work span for the next appointment.

After the initial polishing experiences it is reasonable to progress to a simple buccal pit cavity preparation and restoration. Unless the patient is having pain from very carious teeth, extensive excavations should be avoided in the initial stages. It is surprising how much a small discrete amalgam can inspire a child's confidence and he should be praised for his help in accomplishing the result.

If the operator is called away from the chairside for urgent reasons, the child's confidence may begin to evaporate. It is important on such occasions that the child is never left alone, but the chairside nurse should take over the focus of attention by asking the child, when appropriate, to rinse out, arrange cotton rolls or fix in a different saliva ejector. This type of activity is designed to be complementary to the active dental procedures and should not be confused with chairside 'games' recommended by some operators to take the child's mind off dentistry. Such attempts are only successful until the moment arrives when operative procedures must begin. No child is deceived by such play, which leads to the loss of his confidence in the dentist. The patient knows that he has come to the surgery for dental treatment and it is the operator's task to transform the situation into acceptable terms by means of a carefully graded and sympathetic introduction.

Praise is always a positive form of communication and it has value not only in establishing the child's confidence in the dentist but also in allowing the patient to recruit his self-esteem, a factor of considerable importance for those who have a history of being difficult to treat. No matter how insignificant the success during the visit, the operator should search the situation carefully for some conduct factor that he can praise in front of the waiting parent. For true valour in the chair a certificate of merit signed by the dental nurse can be a source of real pride for those who have tried hard.

Unless there is pain or dental sepsis present the extractions of very carious teeth should be left until the restorative treatment has been completed. This arrangement will allow the thorough assessment of any 'doubtful' teeth which may eventually have to be included in the extraction schedule.

The Uncooperative Child

Children may be uncooperative because they are physically or mentally unable to participate (see Chapter 6) in their treatment. Included in this group are those whose emotional status is so immature that they cannot face the 'up hill' paths of life without considerable support. Children who fall into any of these groups have a history of failure to cooperate and their mouths may show evidence of this with a high caries rate and many attempts at temporary dressings. Another group of patients, however, become uncooperative after a period of successful dental relationships. This 'falling off' may be the result of:

1. Lack of parental concern and personal disillusionment.
2. Alterations in child's emotional environment, e.g. at home where parental separation may have occurred or the arrival of a new baby may make the child feel deprived of parental affection.
3. The most potent factor is fear—fear of pain which the child will not be able to control, and for which he feels he is unable to accept a local anaesthetic. He also fears that the dental surgeon will not know when he is being hurt and that he will continue even when he does. The child is asked to sit in the chair and submit himself to unpleasant and usually lengthy and painful procedures. When all this comes from a person he scarcely knows, it is not surprising that he finds the situation overwhelming. Many fears are augmented by tales at school and children are often remarkably quick to pick upon those who can be easily frightened.

The problem is not to be solved by changing dentists, merely to arrive at the same point of 'impasse'. What is really required is a change of attitudes on the part of the child and dentist and the first point should be based upon an improvement of communication to a level where both can recognise the nature of the problem. The mother may not always be able to help in getting to the root of the child's inability to accept treatment, perhaps because she is too emotionally involved in the patient's behaviour patterns. Such a relationship often makes objective assessment difficult and it is not surprising to find that outside the surgery, the mother may not even discuss with her child his reluctance to accept treatment. Following a wasted appointment, the embarrassment and annoyance which she may show when taking away her uncooperative child, effectively blocks the communication which would help her to appreciate his problems. Her annoyance may be due, in part at least, to the recognition of her own inadequacy in dealing with the situation, whereas her real failure is in her inability to determine the nature of the problem. In these circumstances, therefore, her reaction at the child's lack of coooperation may be one of self-defence. Greater discussion between parent and dentist helps to put the problem in perspective, because in this situation the adult will need as much advice and encouragement as the child.

The relationship between the dentist and his young patient is a delicate one and should be based on the understanding that the operator will make great efforts to explain the nature of the work entailed, and to reduce discomfort to acceptable levels. This may mean reducing considerably the operating programme in order to keep in communication with the patient.

The surgery arrangement already described should receive attention so as to reduce disturbing factors during the introduction of the uncooperative child. Before treatment, the operator should discuss events which have caused lack of cooperation previously, whether at an earlier visit or at another practice. It may have been due to a mistaking of what appeared to be a highly cooperative mood where advantage or urgency caused the dentist to press ahead too quickly with operative techniques. The solution to this problem lies in extending the communication with the child during treatment, stopping frequently to describe the steps being taken and asking the child about those procedures which he finds unpleasant. Sometimes individual factors may cause the child distress, but a sympathetic dental nurse can often choose the moment, when the dentist is away from the chair, to become the child's ally and find what things are upsetting him. With this information the dentist should discuss them openly; do everything possible to eliminate them and then arrange for pain-recognition signals, e.g. raising the hand, so that confidence and trust can be established. Providing sympathy and consideration are shown to apprehensive children they soon realise that dentistry can be an acceptable social experience. Loss of cooperation during a course of dental treatment, especially after a relatively uneventful dental history suggests that extraneous factors may be responsible. These may be emotional in origin and operating at home or school, but deterioration in the child's general health may also make him feel unfit for dental treatment. Whichever factor is involved the dentist must review his own position continually and remember that he has to stay in communication with his patient and not lose his confidence by forcing the issue over one tooth. As a temporary measure during the difficult phase the emphasis of treatment can be changed, e.g. to prophylactic measures or topical application of fluoride, until confidence has been sufficiently re-established to return to schedule. If, however, operative treatment is urgently required as in the case of pulp treatment following traumatic injuries, or the drainage of an acute abscess, recourse may have to be made to a general anaesthetic if the patient is uncooperative.

The anxious child may require premedication and for such cases trimeprazine tartrate (Vallergan) may be given orally as follows:

> For two and a half to seven years of age: Vallergan forte syrup.
> *Dose*: 2-4 mg per kg body weight, one hour before operation.

In the older child trimeprazine may be given the night before, followed by intravenous diazepam at the time of dental treatment. The latter is an effective anxiolytic agent which also confers a retrograde amnesia. However, it does not induce either anaesthesia or analgesia so that routine local anaesthetics must also be used for any painful procedures. The dosage is 0·2 mg per kg body weight, so that a twelve-year-old child would receive a total of approximately 8-10 mg given slowly into a vein of the antecubital fossa. An hour's recovery in the supine position is required afterwards and the child must be supervised for the rest of the day to prevent accidents during the amnesic period. The advantages of such a technique are that the patient retains consciousness but forgets the unpleasant episodes of treatment.

Local Anaesthesia in Children

Equipment layout

1. Spencer-Wells or similar artery forceps at hand in case the needle breaks and there is an opportunity of grasping the fractured end.
2. Hibitane aqueous solution (0·05 per cent) for surface use as antiseptic.
3. Surface anaesthetic either in form of spray or ointment.

4. Disposable syringe with sharp correct length needles.
5. Local anaesthetic solution (containing 1 : 80,000 adrenalin), warmed to blood temperature.
6. Cotton rolls and 'Dry guards'.

Age

By six years of age the use of local anaesthesia can become an accepted procedure if the correct persuasive methods have been used. Some children may be fearful because of previous hospital experiences and in the young there may be the fear of 'going to sleep' and perhaps of separation from the mother. Sympathetic explanations will help the child to realise that he is 'going to stay awake' and it is the gum only which is going to sleep. It is helpful if such terms as 'needle', 'injection', and 'pain' can be avoided and also if the syringe can be kept out of sight beforehand.

Selection and preparation of site

Up to the age of seven years, labial or buccal infiltration of the solution will produce a localised anaesthesia for any teeth except $\overline{6}/6$, which will require an inferior dental nerve block. If the injection can be made in a site prepared by surface anaesthesia a great deal of the discomfort can be reduced and the patient achieves confidence in the technique. Surface anaesthetics should always be used, but even the flavoured variety has to be given with care to prevent it contacting the tongue where it will cause unpleasant anaesthetic sensations. For purposes of confining the liquid and controlling tongue movements cotton rolls, dental napkins or 'Dry guards' should be used on the lingual aspect of the injection site. Two minutes should be given for the surface anaesthetic to become effective, after which the area is cleansed with 0·05 per cent aqueous hibitane solution to remove surface contamination.

Technique for injection

It is necessary to have a clear idea of anatomical structures in the area before giving the injection. Some operators prefer to inject with the left or right hand depending on which side is being anaesthetised, whilst others, use the same hand for both sides. For buccal infiltration, the cheek is gently grasped between thumb and first two fingers so that as it is pulled taut; a firm tent forms in the sulcus which will allow easy entry of the needle. The syringe, its

needle still covered with its disposable sheath, is brought up into
position, its sheath removed and 1·0 ml given slowly into the site.
A little practice allows this action to be completed almost without
the patient's being aware of it and they are surprised to find that
the injection is already accomplished. It is a help with apprehensive
children if the operator can talk continually whilst he is carrying
through his technique, since it serves to refocus the child's attention
away from the site.

Infiltration injections are frequently required for endodontia
procedures on 21/12. The difficulty of obtaining depth of anaesthesic
has been attributed to factors such as the nature of the nerve supply
to the area which may include aberrant nerve branches. The method
recommended is to give a labial infiltration of 1·0 ml of solution
slowly and to wait two minutes before testing for depth of anaesthesia. If any sensation other than touch is still present, it may be
necessary to inject a small quantity of solution into the papilla
distal to the tooth under treatment. Further persistence of sensation, especially in 1/1, can nearly always be overcome by a slow
palatal infiltration directly through the incisive papilla into the
incisive canal, but this is often painful unless great gentleness is
used.

Lower permanent incisors may be anaesthetised by first giving an
injection in the labial sulcus and after a two-minute interval, a
supporting infiltration in the area where the lingual mucosa reflects
on to the inner aspect of the mandible.

The inferior dental block is suitable for children of seven years
and over and is technically more difficult to administer because of
the anatomical field through which the needle passes. In addition
to this the close proximity of the area to the tongue makes the use of
surface anaesthetics less successful. The technique for giving the
injection depends on good initial localisation of the point of entry
for the needle and in order to obtain this the thumb or forefinger is
placed in the retromolar triangle where the stylo-mandibular ligament can be palpated as a ridge on its lingual aspect. Bearing in
mind that the position of the lingula, which is the main deposit area
for the local anaesthetic solution, is at a slightly lower level in
children as compared with adults, the needle is entered at the tip of
the thumb to pass between the lingual and medial aspect of body of
the mandible. A few drops are deposited in this area before the
needle is advanced approximately half an inch in a line with the
dental arch until it contacts the surface of the lingula. It is then withdrawn fractionally, and the direction of the syringe barrel re-aligned
to the opposite canine area so that the needle point slides over the

lingula and the solution is deposited slowly in the area of the neuro-vascular bundle entering the inferior dental canal. It is not necessary to give a buccal infiltration unless extractions are being undertaken. The operator should make it a golden rule during the administration of an inferior dental injection never to remove his guide thumb from the site until the procedure has been completed. If it is maintained there, it keeps the mouth open and compresses the tissues so that if the needle should break there may be an opportunity to grasp the broken end with forceps before it is drawn into the tissues. The reasons for needle breakage are discussed later in this section.

Complications

Haemophilia is the major medical condition which contraindi-cates absolutely the injection of a local anaesthetic solution since enlarging haematomata form within the tissues and are almost impossible to control by normal means. The accumulation of blood following an inferior dental block can increase to such proportions as to cause pressure in the paralaryngeal tissues and produce respira-tory embarrassment which is not amenable to surgical relief such as tracheotomy. Local anaesthesia should also be avoided where there is a low platelet count. There are a number of other situations where precautions are necessary and these are needed if inflammatory processes are present at the injection site. Injection into such sites causes pain and spreads infection so that it is desirable to try regional anaesthesia or to produce anaesthesia in the area by injecting more proximally along the course of the nerve.

If a severe facial cellulitis is present it is inadvisable to use local anaesthesia in any form, not only because of the risk of spreading infection, already mentioned, but also because an accompanying trismus may make an accurate regional anaesthesia technique an uncertain process. The bacteriological status of the tissues can be of profound importance in cases of rheumatic fever and other heart conditions. When there is any risk of introducing bacteria and breaking down natural tissue barriers, the appropriate antibiotic precautions should be taken before hand (see Chapter 6).

Dry sockets rarely occur following extractions with local anaes-thetic in childhood although infection can become a problem if the clot is disturbed whilst anaesthesia is still present. Normally these situations soon improve with hot salt mouthwashes and aspirin, but if the child suffers from diabetes mellitus his tissue resistance to infection is poor and he should receive prophylactic antibiotics (see Chapter 6).

Allergy. If one takes into account the number of dental injections carried out each day, it is remarkable that there are so few allergic reactions to the anaesthetic solution. When it does occur the speed of the reaction can be alarming and is often characterised by an extensive swelling due to escape of tissue fluid into the soft tissue spaces. Following an injection in the upper labial sulcus there may be an extensive oedema of the orbital tissues so that the patient cannot open his eyelids. In such circumstances it may be necessary to arrange for antihistamine therapy as soon as possible and to change the type of anaesthetic solution in the future. Cold compresses and icepacks will improve the condition locally. Allergy is a serious matter and appropriate precautions should be prominently noted on the treatment chart.

Pain. Pain results when the local anaesthetic fluid is injected into inflamed areas, but one of the commonest causes is too rapid delivery of the solution especially where the tissues are closely bound to the bone. The use of disposable syringes and needles means that blunt points are rare although each syringe should be checked before use. The correct manipulation of the tissues should be carried out to make them firm so that the needle penetration can be accomplished easily, otherwise the mucosa will be dragged along before penetration occurs. As already stated it is advantageous to deposit a small amount of local anaesthetic, immediately before manipulating the needle into its required position.

Poor anaesthetic. Whilst poor or short duration anaesthesia may be due to insufficient volume of injected liquid, it is more often due to a failure in technique or releasing the solution in the wrong anatomical position. Most commonly this occurs when giving an inferior dental nerve block, especially if the patient becomes uncooperative.

Fractured needles. There are several factors which contribute to this emergency during injections and they include:

Metallurgic faults in the needle only rarely occur, but it is important in case of legal repercussion to retain carefully the parts of the syringe.

Incorrect length of needle. If the needle is too short and is inserted to the hub, it constitutes a weak site at which it is likely to fatigue by bending. Two other disadvantages from this position are that the rest of the needle cannot be seen and if its fracture occurs there is little opportunity to grasp the end projecting from the tissues with Spencer-Wells forceps.

Incorrect positioning technique when seeking the correct anatomical plane for injection. This may require excessive needle manipulation to find the lingula and causes fatigue of the metal of the needle, usually close to the hub.

Self injury. Where young children are inexperienced in local anaesthesia sensations they are frequently tempted to chew their lips as long as anaesthesia is present (Fig. 1.1). The operator should warn the parents and child against this chewing habit and also the danger from hot foods until normal sensation returns.

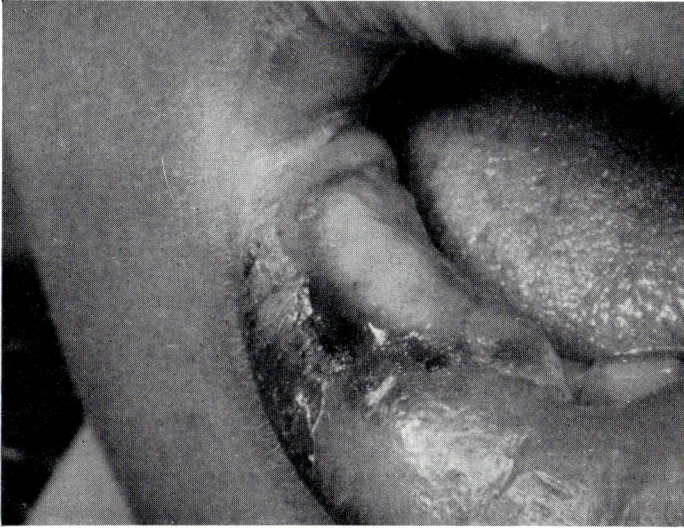

FIG. 1.1. Injury caused by the child chewing the lower lip whilst it was anaesthetised.

Preparation for Simple Surgery Techniques

From a practical point of view many simple surgical procedures including extractions, apicectomy, removal of buried canines and exposure of unerupted teeth can be carried out in the chair using local anaesthesia from eleven years onwards. Before this age it may be necessary to carry out these procedures under general anaesthesia.

Both clinical and radiographic assessment as detailed in Chapter 2 are essential before committing the patient for surgical procedures. The premedication will have to be decided, together with antibiotic cover where extensive flaps and bone removal are envisaged.

Legal Status

The child is a minor until sixteen years of age and must have parental permission before treatment can be carried out. Treatment without such consent constitutes a technical assault. Under certain circumstances however, a teacher or relative can act *in loco parentis* where emergency treatment is required, as when a child's mouth is injured in a fall. Even under such circumstances it is advisable, if possible, to delay extractions and treatment involving general anaesthesia until the parents have given their consent. If, because of illness, they cannot accompany their child they should be sent a letter indicating clearly the treatment required and should be asked to write out the consent in their own hand and sign it, or complete a printed form such as shown below (Fig. 1.2). Alteration in the treatment plan may be necessary to fit changing circumstances, but the operator should ensure that the parent is aware of such changes particularly if these involve extractions and a further consent signature should be obtained.

Soft tissue injuries often accompany dental trauma and where these occur in gardens or agricultural land they should be regarded with suspicion because of the risk of tetanus infection. The organisms responsible for this infection are found in faeces of herbivora and are likely to thrive in torn or lacerated tissues extensively deprived of their normal vascular supply. Where such a risk is thought to exist the dental surgeon should refer the patient for antitetanic toxoid as soon as possible, but if no such facilities are available he should ensure that the patient receives a course of penicillin in adequate dosage. Although there is some dispute concerning the risk of a reaction to the antitetanic serum, the operator should be able to show that he has arranged for his patient to obtain such expert advice as is available.

Instruments and teeth may break during operative procedures and on other occasions a child may struggle so that injuries occur in the mouth before instruments can be removed. It is recognised that such events can occur without there being any question of negligence on the part of the operator who has taken all reasonable precautions. If the dentist is recently qualified he should always attempt to obtain help and advice from more experienced colleagues and should avoid making any comment to parent or child, especially concerning liability, until he has fully assessed the situation. Dressings or sutures may be required for the injured area, or if, for example, a root remains following attempted extractions, the child may need further radiographs to evaluate the situation. Broken needles, instruments and their parts should be retained for metallurgic investigation in case of structural defects. At the same time it is advisable for the operator to contact his professional protection society with details of the incident. The parent must be informed if an injury has occurred

CONSENT TO OPERATION FOR A MINOR

I ....
(Name of Parent or Guardian)

of ....
(Address of Parent or Guardian)

hereby consent to the submission of my child ....to the operation

of ....the effect and nature of which has
been explained to me.

I also consent to such further or alternative operative measures as may be found to be necessary during the course of such operation and to the administration of a local or other anaesthetic for the purpose of the same. I understand that an assurance has not been given that the operation will be performed by a particular surgeon.

Dated this..day of..

Parent or Guardian: ....

Witness : ....
(Signature)
....
(Signature)

....
(Address)

Patient's Case No. ....

FIG. 1.2. Printed consent form.

or if root fragments remain and they should be told what measures, including follow-up procedures, have been arranged to deal with the situation.

The law takes into account the following points when negligence is being considered:

Reasonable forethought and planning (case history)
Proper judgement
Proper degree of skill and care.

2 Case Assessment

A case assessment is a statement of the immediate dental status based on a background of the medical and dental history. It envisages the treatment of specific conditions in a way compatible with related circumstances and makes a reasoned forecast as to the future dental health. More than this, it is a description of facts which may be disputed in law so that information should be included only after a critical review as to its accuracy and completeness.

A suggested scheme for case assessment is shown below. It is followed in detail where it is relevant to each case under consideration.

Age
Present complaint
Medical history
Dental history (including diet)
Dental examination:
1. Inspection of facial contours
2. Preliminary inspection of complaint area
3. Assessment of individual teeth for the following:
    Caries
    Fractures
    Vitality
    Restorations
    Soft tissues, gingival and periodontal conditions
    Attrition, abrasion and erosion
    State of cleanliness
    Stains
    Hypoplasia
    Common developmental abnormalities
4. Assessment of jaw movements
5. Assessment of incisor relationships
6. Assessment of crowding
7. Assessment of skeletal pattern
8. Assessment of function and morphology of soft tissues including tongue, lips and cheeks
9. Detailed examination of complaint
10. Provisional diagnosis and special investigations
11. Case analysis, treatment plan and prognosis

Age

Age is not an accurate guide to morphological development for it has been established that skeletal, chronological and dental ages all progress independently. An example of the use of developmental knowledge is in the treatment of exposed pulps in the fractured 1/1. At approximately eleven years, the apices of 1/1 are completely formed so that there is a good prognosis for a root filling following pulp extirpation. Three years prior to this the apex is incomplete with a wide canal and funnel-shaped apex unsuitable for the standard root filling (Fig. 2.1). From an orthodontic point of view, treatment must be based on the knowledge of developmental horizons. The whole eruption sequence is a calendar in which the units are closely

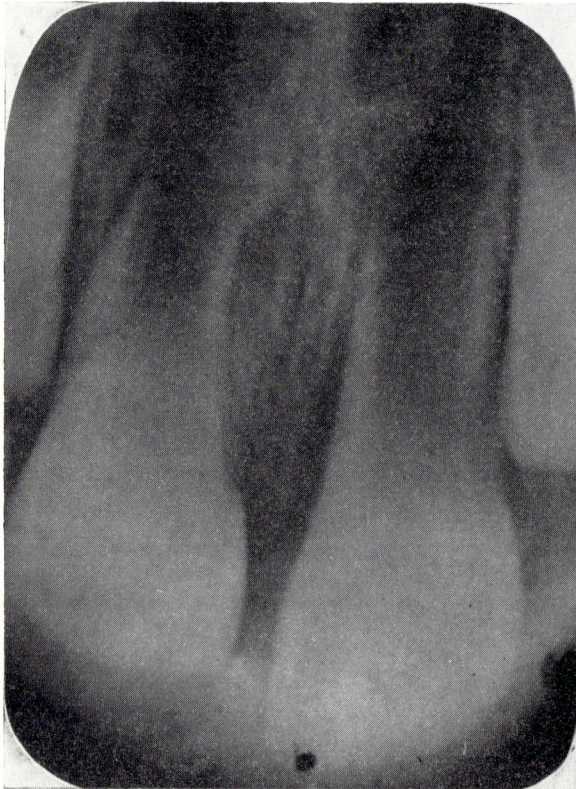

Fig. 2.1. Radiograph showing funnel-shaped root canals of immature permanent central incisors.

interdependent in terms of space allocation and interdigitation. If there is a failure of any part to complete its eruption schedule, an imbalance in the occlusion may result.

Complaint

In this section the comments should be confined to those made by the patient as far as possible. Essentially it is a statement as to why the patient is attending the surgery and may be unrelated to other coexisting oral pathology of which the patient is unaware. Although details of the complaint are left until the section on dental history, these preliminary remarks are useful as a guide in making the assessment. The treatment should be related to the complaint, although the patient must be advised if any other condition requires attention.

Medical History

Two significant aspects which affect dentistry are: (a) How will his medical condition affect his dental treatment, e.g. mongolism? (b) How will dentistry affect his medical condition, e.g. the child with rheumatic heart disease needing extractions? The information should be sought through a general approach by questioning the parent, 'Has your child received any medical care?' or 'Has your child been into hospital?' The information must also include current treatment and take into account drugs which the patients may be receiving. If there is a history of a serious medical condition or if the history is in any way doubtful, with unexplained episodes of illness, the dental surgeon should contact the general medical practitioner for information and advice.

Drugs which affect dental health and treatment

Many drugs are taken for their general action but may produce adverse local reactions such as gingival hyperplasia with phenytoin anticonvulsant treatment. Tooth discoloration will occur where tetracyclines are given to combat infection during the tooth formative periods. Steroids are given to reduce inflammatory reactions and may be prescribed in case of asthma. However, the tissues become more liable to infection, and adrenal shock may occur unless the conditions at operation are carefully regulated. The young diabetic child also requires careful precautions against infection (see Chapter 6) and effective blood sugar control with insulin and diet before general anaesthesia and surgical treatment.

If the work is extensive, preliminary antibiotics and hospital supervision are necessary and should be followed by an adequate supportive programme.

Severe reactions can occur as a result of drug allergies which may include penicillin, procaine and even root canal medicaments, and wherever these are present they require identification and avoidance together with prominent warnings in the case sheets. In an attempt to make treatment more acceptable, anxiolytic drugs such as diazepam are often given either orally or intravenously to the uncooperative patient. It is intended that, under the influence of this drug, these patients shall not lose consciousness and with the help of local anaesthetics they will be able to receive all routine forms of dental treatment. Afterwards the child remembers none of the unpleasant episodes because the drug induces a retrograde amnesia, a factor which the accompanying parent must be aware of, so that the patient can be protected from physical injury by wandering heedlessly into traffic.

When details of medical history have been collected the dental surgeon must decide whether the patient is now fit for treatment which may involve local or general anaesthesia or whether further investigations are necessary.

General Dental History

The operator will have an opportunity to assess the interest and cooperation of parent and child whilst determining the character and extent of previous dental treatment. He will be especially interested where there have been mouth injuries, or difficulty with bleeding or healing following extractions under local or general anaesthesia. In the case of trauma received during car accidents the child may be the subject of litigation which might well depend upon evidence from current observations made by the dental surgeon of the extent of dental injuries and their prognosis. The child may be receiving orthodontic treatment concurrently, in which case further communication will be necessary to determine the relevant history and future plans.

If the patient has been seen recently by other dental practitioners the operator should review this aspect of the history carefully, for it may reveal that the child is currently under the care of another dental surgeon but has refused to accept his treatment. In other cases this type of history may indicate that the child has been uncooperative during treatment or that there has been poor support from the parents in keeping appointments.

It is essential that the dental history should include information on toothbrushing habits and diet both as regards detersive foods and those containing refined carbohydrates such as biscuits (see Chapter 3).

History of present complaint

The general comments made by the patient must now be supplemented by accurate and detailed information concerning the exact nature of the disturbance, e.g. pain, its duration, extent, exciting and relieving factors together with associated features such as swelling or discoloration.

Dental Examination

Inspection of facial contours

Although few faces are truly symmetrical, examination of their contours is important because it may reveal swellings of non-dental origin, besides those due to the spread of infection from oral tissue. It may also be a help in indicating the degree to which skeletal factors may effect malocclusion.

Preliminary inspection

Examination of the complaint area usually indicates the general nature of the dental problem and if this is acute it may require urgent treatment. However it is necessary to make an assessment of the other areas of the mouth since a similar situation may be present elsewhere although asymptomatic. Such a case often arises with very carious lower 1st permanent molars where both teeth can be extracted in the same schedule if a general anaesthetic is to be given. Whatever the complaint, the patient will expect to have it put right or at least improved as a result of treatment. In assessing the dental tissues it is important to realise that the order of examination is not rigidly fixed—and should be governed by the nature of the complaint.

If the time making the full assessment is to be efficiently used, it is a great advantage to have radiographic evidence available whilst the tissues are being examined. The preliminary inspection serves as a useful stage for determining what radiographs will be necessary for the complete examination. The views required are periapicals in traumatic dental injuries, full mouth bitewings for caries, or in the case of a malocclusion an orthopantomograph of the

B

jaws plus periapical views of $\dfrac{3—/—3}{3—/—3}$; occlusal views will be required
if canine positions are in doubt.

Dental models will be required for the assessment where the patient has an orthodontic problem and impressions for these can be taken conveniently during the preliminary inspection stage.

Once these arrangements have been carried out, the operator can take advantage of the additional diagnostic information which will be available during the assessment.

Assessment of individual teeth

The teeth should be counted and surveyed systematically in a good light, referring in each instance to the bitewing and periapical radiographs. If the patient has periodontal problems it may be preferable to make the assessment of these tissues and the state of tooth cleanliness before the caries estimation. The reason for this order of examination is that an effective caries assessment cannot be made without first carrying out a thorough dental prophylaxis.

Caries

It is of interest, before discussing caries detection, to note the average patterns of caries experience in children.

Primary dentition: percentage of children with caries

By 1 yr	5% have caries
By 2 yr	15% have caries
By 3 yr	40% have caries
By 4 yr	55% have caries
By 5 yr	75% have caries

Average caries-extent in primary teeth in terms of decayed and filled surfaces (D.F.S.)

By 2 yr	0·3 D.F.S.
By 3 yr	1·0 D.F.S.
By 4 yr	2·5 D.F.S.
By 5 yr	4·6 D.F.S.

After 8 yr: D.F.S. rise to 8·0

Relative caries susceptibility of primary teeth. By the age of two years approximately 60 per cent of caries is occlusal with only insignificant proximal molar caries. In the incisors 25 per cent of the caries is proximal. However, by the age of six years the occlusal and proximal caries rates are equal, and it is thought that initially independent factors may influence the development of each type of lesion.

The 1st primary molars are less susceptible to caries than the 2nd primary molars. It is not, therefore, surprising to find the eight-year-old child with 50 per cent of the 2nd primary molars carious, whereas only 20 per cent of the 1st primary molars are affected. Similarly, if there is distal caries of the 1st primary molar then one may expect a mesial lesion on the relevant 2nd primary molar.

Relative susceptibility of 1st permanent molars to contact caries from 2nd primary molars. Usually by six years of age there are ten times more caries on the mesial of the 2nd primary molars than on their distal surfaces. Three years later the distal surface of this tooth has nearly half as much caries as the mesial area. Generally there is a much more moderate caries attack on the mesial of the 1st primary molar.

Caries in the permanent dentition. The eruption of all permanent teeth except the 3rd molars is usually completed by fourteen years of age.

Permanent dentition: percentage of children with caries

By 6 yr	20% have caries
By 8 yr	60% have caries
By 10 yr	85% have caries
By 12 yr	90% have caries

Average caries extent in permanent teeth in terms of D.M.F.

By 6 yr	0·5 D.M.F.
By 8 yr	2·4 D.M.F.
By 10 yr	3·7 D.M.F.
By 12 yr	5·9 D.M.F.

D = teeth decayed.
M = teeth extracted because of caries.
F = teeth filled.

In practical terms these figures indicate that a new cavity appears in the dentition for each year of eruption of permanent teeth.

In terms of decayed, missing and filled surfaces (D.M.F.S.) of permanent teeth

By 6 yr D.M.F.S. score = D.M.F. score (i.e. 2·4)
By 12 yr D.M.F.S. score = 7·5

Order of caries attack. Up to twelve years, mainly the 1st permanent molars are affected in the following way:

By 7 yr	25% of $\overline{6|6}$ become carious
By 9 yr	50% of $\overline{6|6}$ become carious
By 12 yr	70% of $\overline{6|6}$ become carious
By 7 yr	12% of $6|6$ are affected
By 9 yr	35% of $6|\overline{6}$ are affected
By 12 yr	52% of $6|\overline{6}$ are affected

$21|\overline{12}$ *are less susceptible to caries*

At 8 yr	1% of these are carious
At 11 yr	10% of these are carious
At 12 yr	15% of these are carious

Caries in $\overline{21|12}$ is minimal so that by twelve years of age only 2 per cent are affected. If, therefore, proximal caries is present in these teeth, the prognosis is poor unless effective control measures can be adopted right away.

The average caries experience in premolars shows that in the twelve-year-old, 5·0 per cent of $\dfrac{54|45}{5|5}$ are affected. However the 2nd permanent molars which erupt at twelve years are caries-susceptible, so that 20 per cent of $\overline{7|7}$ and 10 per cent of $7|\overline{7}$ show caries within a year of eruption.

Caries susceptibility of various surfaces of permanent teeth. Between six and twelve years, occlusal cavities are most frequent, and occur in the molars shortly after eruption, and proximal caries in the posterior teeth usually follows.

By twelve years 50 % of caries in permanent molars is occlusal,
30 % is proximal,
20 % is buccal and ligual.
Less than 1 % is labial, incisal or cervical.

The 1st permanent molars are the most caries-susceptible of all the permanent teeth.

By 6 yr 62 % of children show fissure caries
By 7 yr 76 % of children show fissure caries
By 8 yr 94 % of children show fissure caries

Mesial caries in these teeth:

> By 6 yr 2 % of these children were affected
> By 7 yr 5 % of these children were affected
> By 8 yr 33 % of these children were affected

Speed of caries. The crowns of primary molars have been known to be destroyed to gum level by caries in less than one year from their eruption. Badly constructed partial dentures and orthodontic appliances can also bring about great carious destruction especially where effective oral hygiene is not practised.

Occlusal caries progresses at a very variable rate, in some cases taking as little as three months to change from incipient caries to a recognisable cavity. On other occasions this process may take as long as four years.

Caries differences between boys and girls. Generally girls show a slightly greater caries experience in their permanent dentition compared with boys, possibly because of the earlier eruption of their teeth. However this difference becomes less, after twelve years of age.

Caries rate of children and their parents. The children whose parents have sound teeth, tend to have less caries-susceptible teeth themselves. On the other hand, parents with severe caries problems may expect their children to have twice as many carious teeth when compared with boys and girls of the former group.

Caries detection. VISION. Obvious cavities in the teeth present no difficult diagnostic task, but careful scrutiny is needed to determine the significance of local loss of crown translucency. Where such changes are associated with the fissure systems of the occlusal surfaces they may indicate that there is a large undermining mass of caries but with a scarcely detectable surface breach. In the proximal regions a similar loss of translucency associated with a slight reciprocal drift of affected teeth indicates that there has been a carious, destruction of the contact points which has allowed such movement to occur. Associated with this type of lesion it is not uncommon to find a history of food packing in the defective area causing damage and pain in the interdental papillae.

In the incisor area proximal caries may be revealed by discoloration or loss of translucency particularly when the teeth are transilluminated with reflected light from the palatal aspect.

Areas of chalky caries which result from the breakdown of the enamel after persistent exposure to a low pH environment usually occur at the cervical margins of the crowns. The distribution of the lesions is usually on the labial surfaces of CBA/ABC, but later the

21/12 (Fig. 2.2) and buccal surfaces 6/6, and both lingual and buccal surfaces of 6/6, become affected. Such lesions may sometimes occur in patients who have worn multiband appliances for a prolonged period without supervision and indicate that they require an urgent reappraisal of both their orthodontic rationale and also the mouth hygiene. The significance of this problem is discussed in Chapter 8.

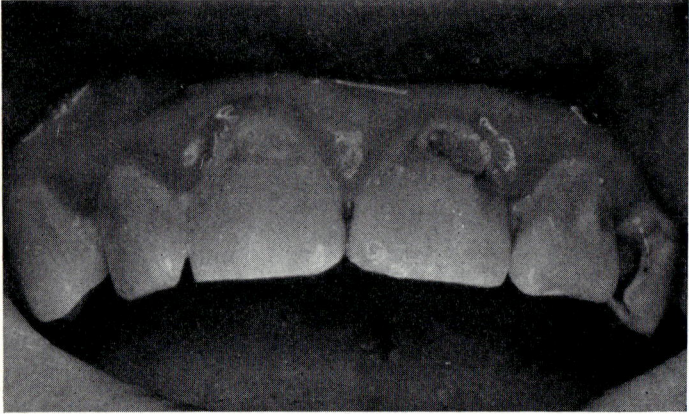

FIG. 2.2. Cervical caries of 21/12 in a mouth showing neglect and stagnation.

An improvement in the oral environment is seen in mouths with arrested caries. These usually occur in the primary dentition and, although the teeth are discoloured, the enamel peripheral to the lesion has broken down leaving a smooth, saucerised and shallow cavity (Fig. 2.3). No symptoms are associated with these teeth and they normally remain functional and healthy.

THE PROBE POINT. The fine point of the dental probe is one of the most sensitive instruments that the operator has at his disposal. It is a delicate extension of his fingers capable of telling him of remarkably small changes in the texture of hard tissues. The point should be sharp and its shape such that it can investigate the relevant surfaces without interference from adjacent structures. For effective caries assessment the instruments available should include a half-moon, a straight and a Briault probe. Between them they are capable of detecting four basic sensations:

1. *Surface roughness* associated with early chalky caries.
2. *'Sticky fissures.'* The deep anatomical shape of the fissures, sometimes associated with decalcification or active caries of its walls, gives a sticking sensation on probing.

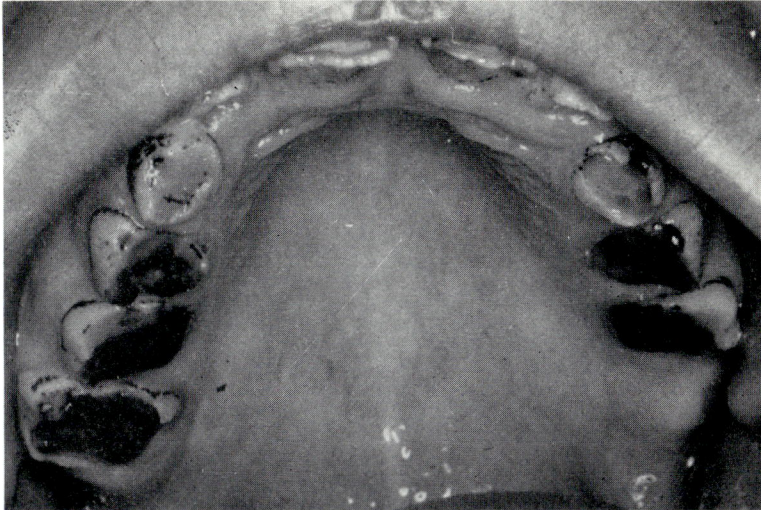

Fig. 2.3. Arrested caries of primary and permanent teeth.

3. *Soft dentine* found within a cavity allows extensive probe penetration and indicates active caries often painful to probing.
4. *Overhanging hard enamel margins* at the rim of a carious lesion
   especially of the interproximal variety. The presence of a
   'catch' infers that a margin is present.

Bitewing radiographs. Five intraoral films are required to
cover the caries investigation (Fig. 2.4).

The cusp superimposition on the film prevents radiographic
detection of all, except large, occlusal cavities. When, however,
the latter are present, their extent in relation to the pulp horns is of
value in assessing the likelihood of a carious exposure. It has to be
emphasised however that caries is always more extensive clinically
than its radiographic appearance indicates so that any deep lesion
must be regarded as a potential threat to the pulp.

Superimposition in proximal crown areas is due either to crowding
and overlapping of teeth or alternatively, to poor tube alignment.
Where the important contact points are shown as discrete structures,
early caries is recognised as a break in the continuity of the enamel
outline (Fig. 2.4). The radiograph will only reveal a rarefied area in
adjacent dentine if the lesion has progressed to a substantial size.
The value of routine bitewing radiographs is emphasised where

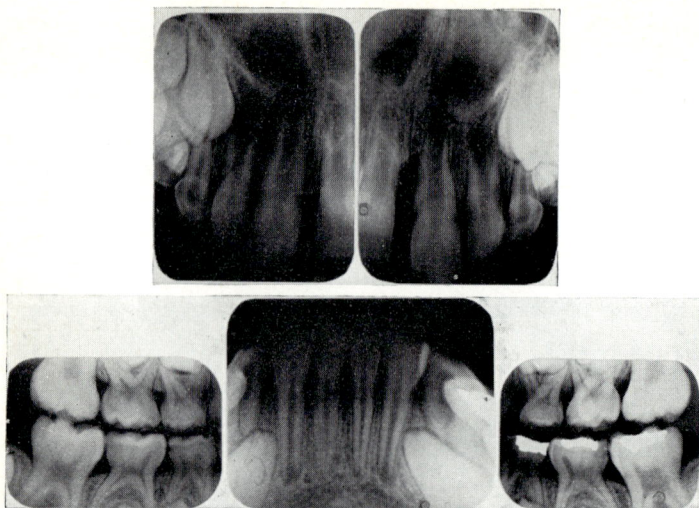

Fig. 2.4. Standard radiographs for caries.

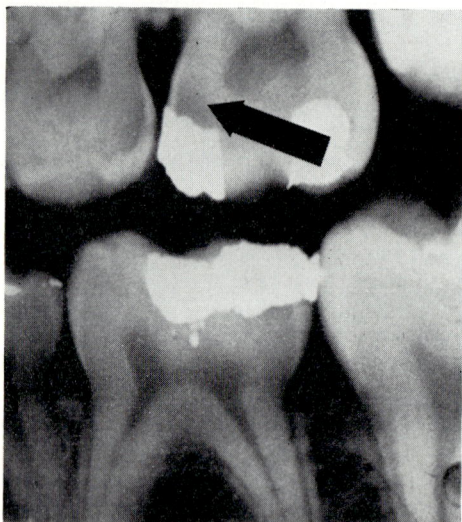

Fig. 2.5. Radiograph showing caries beneath an amalgam restoration.

recurrent caries can sometimes be demonstrated beneath amalgam restorations as a cause of pain (Fig. 2.5).

The caries experience of the individual is usually expressed in terms of the number of teeth decayed; extracted (not for orthodontic reasons); or filled: d.e.f. (primary dentition), D.M.F. (permanent teeth). The D.M.F. (or d.e.f.) figure represents the sum of the scores to give a total of caries experience for each child.

Another method of expressing the severity of the caries experience is to consider the number of surfaces of each tooth affected, the total score being expressed as D.M.F.(S.). By this method each extracted tooth is given a score allocation which is added to the sum of the scores for other teeth. In both these assessment methods, the 'sticky fissure' is often ignored in the scoring for purposes of standard-isation of examination techniques.

Fractures and traumatic injuries

Tooth fracture occurs more easily if the crowns are weakened by hypoplasia, caries, restorations or endodontic treatment. Crown and root fractures are less common in primary teeth following injury but, however, they tend to displace easily due to the greater flexibility of supporting bone and nearby developing permanent teeth. Root resorption progressively decreases their support as they near exfoliation time.

Fractures of the tooth can be classified as follows:

1. Enamel crazing (Fig. 2.6).
2. Enamel fractures.
3. Fractures into dentine.
4. Fractures involving the pulp (Fig. 2.7).
5. Root fracture (Fig. 2.8).
6. Oblique crown-root fractures.

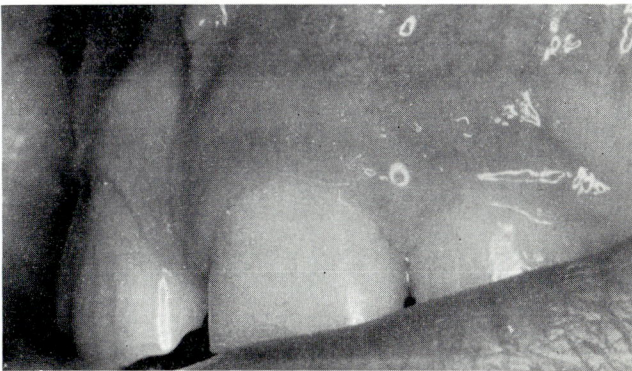

FIG. 2.6. Crazing of injured enamel of 1/1.

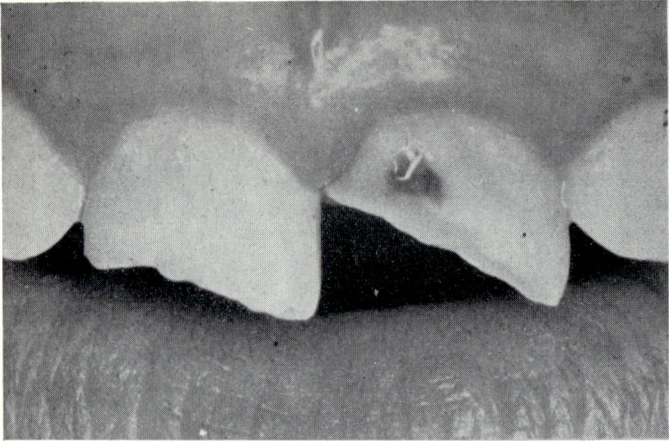

FIG. 2.7. Crown fracture involving the pulp.

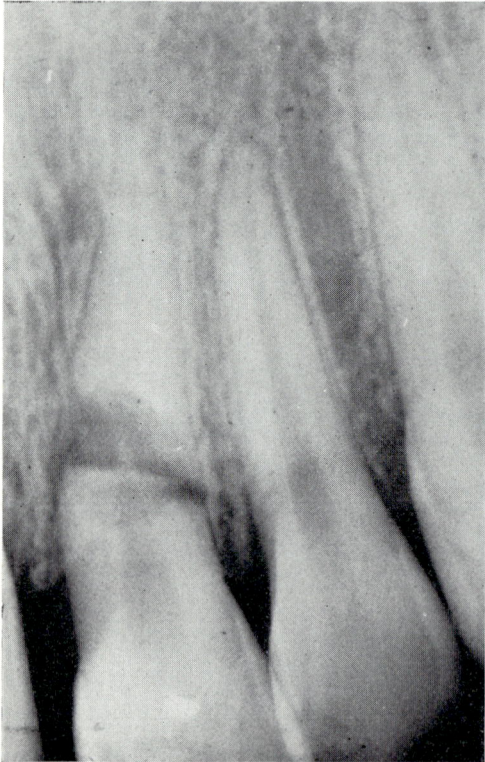

FIG. 2.8. Radiograph of a permanent central incisor with a root fracture.

Clinical assessment of injured teeth involves examination of the following:

1. COLOUR. The crown may be congested with blood or discoloured as a result of pulp necrosis. Such changes are more obvious on transillumination but comparison with adjacent normal teeth will make differences more obvious. Transillumination is also valuable in demonstrating enamel crazing.

2. POSITION. Alteration in incisal levels should be interpreted with care. Such a difference may indicate displacement during trauma, but it may be the result of under-eruption, deflection by thumb-sucking habits or supernumeraries. Like so many investigations in oral trauma, no single factor should be taken in isolation, but conclusions should always be based on as broad a spectrum of evidence as possible.

3. PULP. The position of crown fracture may be deceptive in partly erupted teeth, but direct evidence of pulp exposure should be sought using a sharp probe passed gently over the deeper dentine aspects. A catch in the surface should be viewed with suspicion even if no bleeding occurs, since in this situation the pulp horn may be exposed but necrotic especially if examination has been delayed for over forty-eight hours. Vertical or oblique fractures of the crown may be difficult to detect and great care should be taken to investigate for possibility of separation of all vertical hairline cracks. Careful observation may show a minute oozing of pulp tissue fluid and blood when the sharp probe point is inserted into the line. Pain is a significant feature during this test, but also by keeping a careful eye on the outline of the main fracture plane, one part of the crown can be seen moving relative to the other during the probing. This situation becomes more evident after twenty-four hours when the injured pulp swells and protrudes between the separating fragments of the vertical fracture.

4. PALPATION. The lip is retracted, and the forefinger of the examining hand is gently rested against the incisal edge of each tooth in the affected segment. It is possible to assess the normal degree of mobility of the teeth within the arch at that stage of development, and also to determine if any show a greater range than normal. Increased vertical and rotatory movements commonly found after the tooth has been forced into the bone, indicate extensive rupture of the peridontal ligaments. However, since mobility may also be an indication of root fracture, gentle handling is advised during the assessment of mobility.

5. PERCUSSION. This is carried out by gently tapping the incisor in an axial direction, but is not usually practised immediately after

trauma since the accumulation of blood clot and tissue fluid confuses the result. Later when periodontal reattachment has been allowed to occur, pain on percussion is indicative of increase in periapical pressure often due to a developing dental abscess. Teeth with fractured roots give a different sound on percussion compared with adjacent incisors.

6. RADIOGRAPHS. The type of radiographic examination used in oral injury will depend on the nature and extent of the trauma. If the situation is complicated by facial injury and the possibility of skeletal fractures then the radiographic survey should include all doubtful areas. Orthopantomograph, lateral skull and postero-anterior skull views may be needed to give good views of such features as mandibular condyles and jaw outlines. The orthopanto-mograph may be of value where panoramic jaw views are needed, but once the incisors are included in the injury, the routine periapical views will nearly always give better detail of local disturbances of these teeth and their immediate environment.

Value of preliminary radiograph. 1. It serves as a record of the state of the injured tissues shortly after the accident.

2. It gives basic information concerning the state of development and dental age of the child, e.g. whether the apical formation is completed.

3. Presence of extraneous disease, e.g. abnormal crown structures dens invaginatus, root dilacerations not associated directly with the immediate injury.

4. Evidence of injury to the crown, root and its attachment, periapical and surrounding tissues, and unsuspected injury to adjacent teeth, and presence of root fillings.

5. Soft tissue radiographs may sometimes show radio-opaque objects, e.g. tooth fragments embedded in the lip at the time of injury. In general therefore it is an advantage to obtain radiographic evidence of the injury as soon as possible.

Radiographic evidence of dental injury. An excellent rule for looking at radiographs is to classify the search in relationship to the tissues so that the whole field is systematically surveyed, but first identify the correct viewing side of the radiograph. Similar fractures of 1/1 will lead to error if the appearance of the teeth on the film is used as the criterion for identification.

Systematic examination of radiograph. Superfluous light from the viewing box should be blacked out so that attention can be concentrated on the X-ray field.

CROWN FRACTURES. Direction of fracture is apparent and also its extent in relation to the pulp and root. A vertical fracture of crown is difficult to detect.

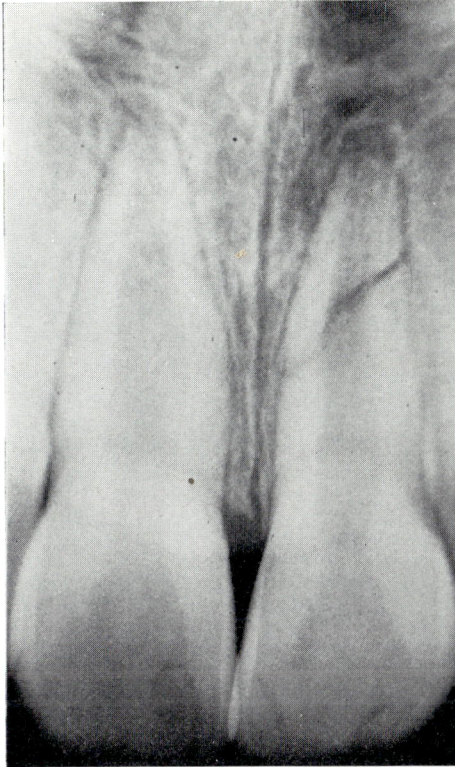

FIG. 2.9. Radiograph of an upper permanent central incisor which demonstrates the 'step' in the outline of the fractured root.

ROOT. Evidence of fracture may not show as a separation of fractured root surfaces. If the fracture plane is parallel to direction of X-rays then the fracture will appear as a single well-defined black line with a step in the outline of the root (Fig. 2.9). Where the fractured plane is oblique to the direction of the X-rays, the palatal and labial aspect of the plane will appear at two different heights on the root and they will also be fainter. The characteristic step in the root outline will also be more difficult to define. It is unusual to find more than one fracture of the same root but adjacent incisors may both have similar radicular fractures.

The position of the root fracture is of major importance in the prognosis and treatment planning and as a general rule the nearer the fracture to the neck of the tooth the poorer the prognosis because crown displacements are much more liable to occur due to reduced attachment. Where such displacement occurs, healing by fibrous or calcific union across the fractured ends in unlikely. When the fracture occurs in the apical third, displacement of the fractured surfaces is less likely and apical root resection can be carried out if root canal treatment becomes necessary.

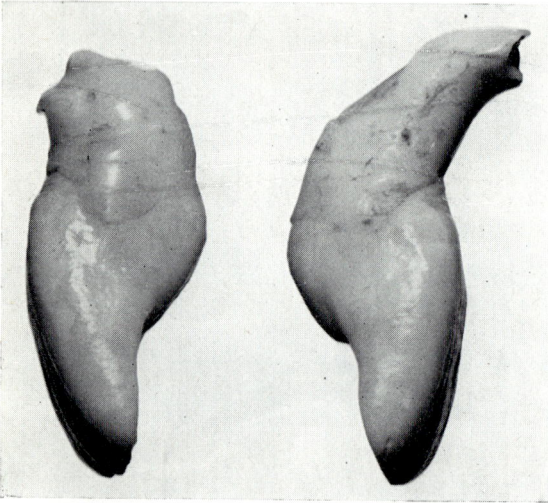

Fig. 2.10 Photograph of the mesial surfaces of surgically removed, unerupted permanent central incisors with dilacerated roots.

Injury to the apical portion of the developing root may be difficult to demonstrate radiographically apart from a loss of the regular funnel-shaped apical outline accompanied by evidence of displacement of the root walls. Later, the developing root may show a dilacerated form (Fig. 2.10) and this might take the form of partial arrest of normal dentine formation (Fig. 2.11). Degenerative changes such as pulp calcification may be in evidence on radiographs of injury to either primary or permanent teeth (Fig. 2.12).

Vertical or oblique fractures of crown and root are difficult to detect radiographically and the best evidence of their presence is usually found by using clinical methods already discussed. Root

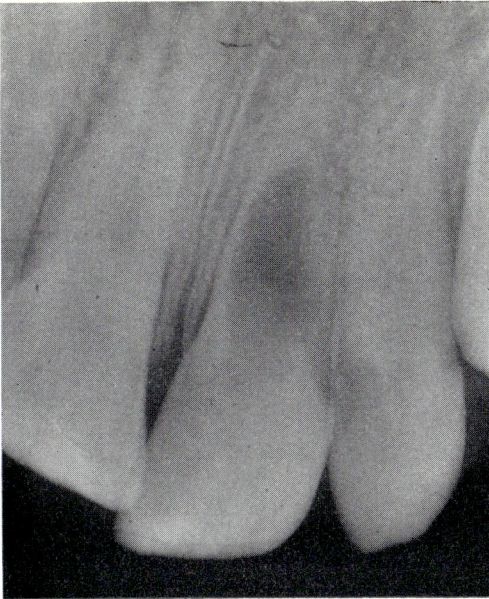

Fig. 2.11. Radiograph of permanent central incisor with arrested root development.

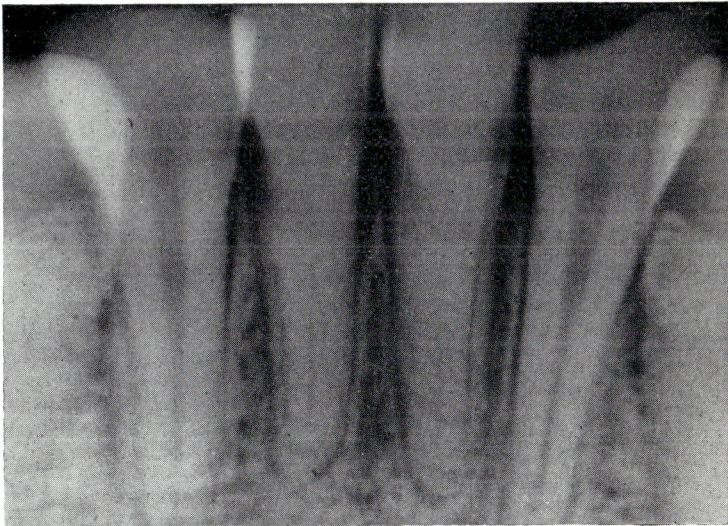

Fig. 2.12. Radiograph showing evidence of degenerative pulp calcification in lower permanent central incisors.

resorption may sometimes follow injury (Fig. 2.13) and also after tooth replantation.

PERIODONTAL LIGAMENT. Whilst the periodontal ligament is not visible on the radiographs, the alteration in the size of the space that it occupies can be useful evidence of its integrity. Violent movements of the root that occur when the tooth is forced out of position result in extensive haemorrhage of the periodontal ligament and sometimes the apical neurovascular bundle is also torn. Injury is followed

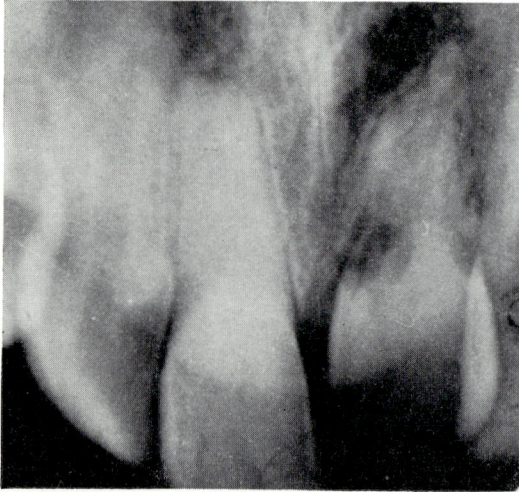

FIG. 2.13. Radiograph indicating root resorption of /1 following a traumatic injury. The adjacent central incisor is also abnormal.

by an inflammatory reaction as a result of which the increase of fluid, blood clot and many torn periodontal fibres produce a partial extrusion of the root from its normal position in the socket. From a radiographic point of view, movement of the tooth out of its socket shows more clearly at the apex than around the lateral aspects of the root, but there is nevertheless an overall well-marked radiolucent margin around the root (Fig. 2.14). A similar picture can be found sometimes in an acute dental abscess resulting from pulp necrosis, although in these circumstances, since most of the periodontal fibres are intact, the accumulating inflammatory pressure around the tooth can find only a limited relief by pushing the tooth out of its socket. A situation then develops where the tooth becomes very tender to the touch, but this is not so in cases where trauma has occurred.

Evidence of periapical injury may relate to changes occurring in the pulp tissue. During trauma the pulp is vulnerable in three respects:

1. From failure of its vascular supply, either completely by severance of the vascular bundle as a result of its shearing between

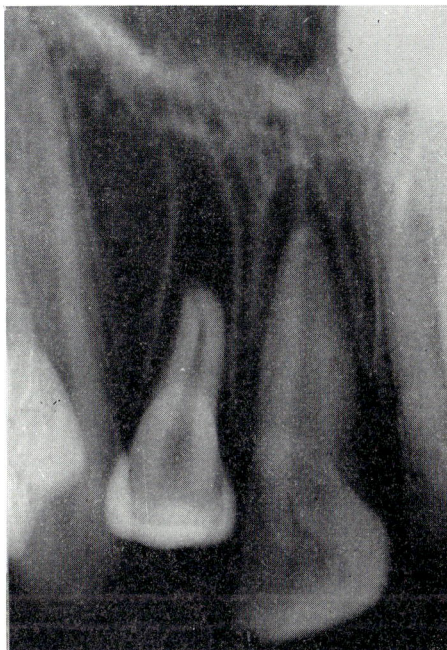

FIG. 2.14. Radiograph showing the appearance of teeth partly displaced from their sockets by trauma. The greater opacity of the 2/ is due to its long axis being tilted more parallel to the X-ray beam.

the hard outer faces of root and socket, or alternatively the apical vessels may be crushed by injury so that the blood supply to the pulp is reduced.

2. Exposure of the pulp horns leading to infection of the tissues or, indirectly, where thermal or chemical irritants lead to pulp hyperaemia.

3. Internal changes occurring within the pulp, initiated possibly by alterations in vascular supply but leading to degenerative changes such as calcification or fibrosis.

The periapical bone is a sensitive indicator of pulp damage, and providing sufficient time is given, it will react to changes in its immediate environment. If the pulp is necrotic or infected, the toxic products of its breakdowns pass into the periapical tissues. When the release of these products is slow, there is a mild stimulating, osteoblastic activity. This is shown on the radiograph as a localised increased bone density around the tooth apex called sclerosing osteitis. The majority of cases, however, demonstrate the more toxic effects of pulp necrosis by the development of well-defined areas of bone loss where osteoclastic activity is the predominant feature (rarefying osteitis). If the pulp breakdown occurs rapidly as with an acute pulpitis and dental abscess, the radiograph shows that the appearance of periapical rarefaction is diffusely related to the apex of the affected tooth, and possesses no well-defined margin to the lesion as one would expect around a more chronic condition.

Pulp vitality

Thermal tests are carried out by isolating the teeth with cotton rolls and gently drying the tooth surfaces. Incisors with fractures into deep dentine may be very sensitive to thermal changes so that when testing, heat and cold should not be applied directly to the dentine surface unless there is no response from other parts of the crown. This is carried out by spraying ethyl chloride on to a pledget of cotton wool which is applied to the labial aspect of adjacent crowns before testing the injured crown. The child should not be told what sensation to expect from the fractured tooth, since anxiety may make him anticipate a hoped-for response. It is an advantage to be able to see the patient's eyes during the testing, since sudden alteration of pupil size indicates his experience of unpleasant sensation. In order to elicit a reasonable response the patient is told 'You can feel me touching the tooth. Can you feel anything else?' The method is applied to adjacent teeth, particularly in following up traumatic injuries where the urgency of replanting a displaced tooth may distract the attention from the possibility of damage to a nearby incisor.

By alternatively applying the refrigerated and non-cooled cotton wool to the test tooth so that the child cannot predict the sequence, it is usually possible to separate his enthusiasm from the genuine pulp sensation.

Heat applied to the fractured tooth is usually by means of heated gutta-percha, but a preliminary smear of vaseline to this crown prevents it sticking during the test. Care should be taken to avoid applying heat directly to the fractured surface and it should be confined to the labial aspect of the crown.

INTERPRETATION OF RESPONSES TO THERMAL CHANGES. Variations in response are great; some patients completely failing to respond to one or both forms of stimulation. If these tests are carried out after eight to ten weeks following injury then a variety of changes may have occurred or be occurring within the pulp tissue. Such changes may be necrotic or degenerative in type, although an early secondary dentine response may account for the reduced response.

If the patient's tooth responds to either heat or cold stimulations, normal vitality may not always be assumed, since heightened sensation with heat may indicate a pulp hyperaemia.

Electrical tests. In the absence of any response to thermal changes, further testing should be carried out using electric testers in the following manner.

The tooth is gently cleansed and isolated and the crown thoroughly dried. Rubber dam is not always practicable when there is an oblique fracture plane, but careful use of cotton rolls and napkins will act as a good substitute if they are maintained in place by the operator during the test. The patient holds the indifferent electrode in one hand and the stimulating electrode point is moistened to establish good electrical conductivity on to the tooth surface, but at the same time the point of application should be as far from the cervical margin as possible and preferably on the fractured surface. The patient is instructed to raise the free hand when tingling is felt in the tooth but the operator should expect that the patient might interpret the sensation as heat, cold, or pain. The voltage is gradually increased until a response is elicited.

INTERPRETATION OF ELECTRICAL PULP-TESTING. Provided that the testing has been carefully carried out, a response usually indicates that the pulp is vital, but misleading results can occur. Very occasionally it is possible to obtain results where the tooth's pain perception threshold value is within the normal range despite the fact that the pulp is almost completely necrotic. On the other hand, high or low readings do not necessarily indicate pulp hyperaemia or pulpitis or degenerative changes.

In general, however, the electrical response of a tooth may be taken as a good guide to its vitality, but too narrow an interpretation is to be avoided and results should always be used in association with a full clinical assessment.

Standards for comparison may be obtained by first testing adjacent or similar teeth in the mouth, a particularly important feature if thermal methods are being used. Decisions are difficult where there is no evidence of periapical pathology either clinically or from the radiograph and yet no response can be obtained from the tests. Guidance in these circumstances can be obtained from determining the response of adjacent teeth to testing. If there is a marked difference between the two series of tests this would increase one's suspicions concerning the tooth under review. However, the presence of many restorations in all the anterior teeth may make this comparative evidence less valuable.

Doubtful pulp vitality in children with rheumatic heart disease is a serious matter (see Chapter 6) and requires early and positive action by the operator. In these cases the tooth should be extracted as soon as possible. The operator is not justified in keeping these cases 'under observation' until more positive dental evidence presents itself.

Under normal circumstances it is not necessary to test the vitality of all teeth in the healthy patient, unless there is a question of detecting the origin of swelling, pain or infection. However, the operator is rightly reserved in his opinion where multisurface restorations are present in molars and premolars or where incisors and canines have been extensively filled with silicate fillings. Periapical radiographic evidence is essential in making a dental assessment in these cases.

Restorations

Restorations are carried out for teeth affected by caries, trauma or with poor aesthetics. In many mouths these conditions may have been treated by intermediate measures in order to allow for developmental changes to occur, e.g. basket crowns. The assessment of the mouth, however, must include a critical appraisal of all restorations present, bearing in mind the following points:

1. Is the restoration functional in such a way that it produces optimal occlusal relationships and prevents overeruption, drift, and alteration of spatial arrangement within the arch?

2. Is the restoration physically adequate to carry out its function? Large Class III cavities may leave the incisal edge too weak to stand mastication, and should be extended to take a Class IV inlay. If mesial and distal surfaces are involved a jacket crown replacement will be superior in strength and appearance with only slight increase in the overall operating time.

3. Is the restoration fulfilling the aesthetic standards? Incisors extensively restored with plastic fillings may be improved if these were replaced by jacket crowns.

4. Is there a risk of pulp injury? Large Class III cavities in young incisors present other problems as well as those mentioned. During extensions of the cavity to obtain as much intracoronal retention as possible pulp exposure may have occurred. Such a breach may not always be evident particularly if local anaesthesia is used, but chronic inflammatory pulp changes usually follow, perhaps undiscovered for several months. Where silicate restorations are inserted in cavities with an inadequately protected pulp, subsequent inflammatory or degenerative changes are very likely to occur. Thus in reviewing old restorations the possibility of either traumatic or chemical injury to the pulp should be borne in mind.

The soundness of a restoration depends upon:

1. *Adequate outline* to prevent recurrence of caries and to allow appropriate cavity design. This factor is essential in Class II restorations of primary molars (see Chapter 3) otherwise amalgam fracture commonly occurs.

2. *Adequate retention form* is essential in jacket crown preparations, particularly in severely fractured incisors (see Chapter 5) where the amount of sound crown available is restricted.

3. *Adequate occlusal replacement.* Failure to restore the contact point will result in food packing and injury to the interdental soft tissues and the possibility of caries recurring on the adjacent proximal tooth surface. Over-restored occlusal surfaces of Class II amalgams may result in a fracture at the isthmus of the proximal extension, traumatic high spots and deviation of the occlusion due to premature and painful contact.

4. *Streamlined contour* of the restoration is important in the economical management of food. Rough margins irritate the tongue and lips and allow food stagnation. Inadequately contoured restorations with positive cervical ledges can cause extensive inflammatory damage of the interdental papilla and underlying tissues resulting in periodontal pocket formation.

5. Materials require *correct preparation* and must be inserted in an *uncontaminated condition.* To satisfy these needs the elimination of saliva and blood during the cavity toilet stage, must receive attention.

Soft tissue, gingival and periodontal conditions

For treatment of these conditions see Chapter 6. Changes in the gingivae may be due to a variety of causes.

Teething. 'Teething' has provided a useful peg on to which many minor disturbances can be hung. These have included transient fevers, fits, coughs, gastro-intestinal disturbances such as diarrhoea and vomiting. Coincidental with many of these features which are fairly common in early childhood, there may be oral signs and symptoms including:

> Pain and swelling over the eruption site and occasionally haematoma formation (Fig. 2.15).
> Salivation and dribbling.
> Digit sucking.
> Sometimes associated herpetiform ulcers in other parts of the mouth.
> Slight halitosis.
> Bright red cheeks.
> Occasionally, enlargement of regional lymph nodes.

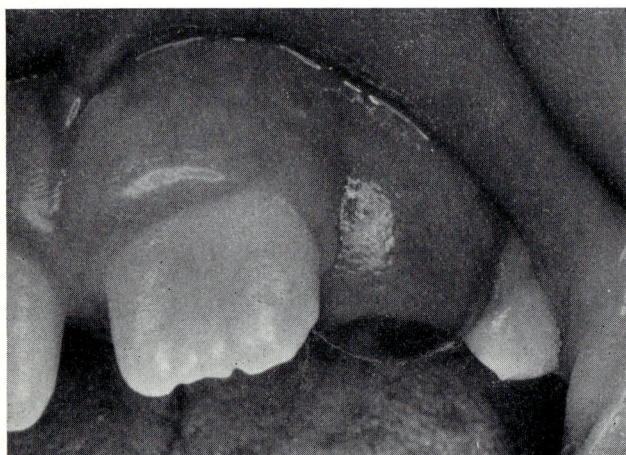

FIG. 2.15. Eruption cyst forming over a permanent lateral incisor.

The interesting feature about tooth eruption is that it does not always happen in a painful manner but it is common for most children to have at least one difficult episode during their two and a half years primary eruption experience. Very occasionally the appearance of 1st permanent molars may also be heralded by local pain and swelling. If due regard is given to many of the general signs and symptoms associated with teething, they are indicative of some form of mild infection, possibly gastro-intestinal or upper respiratory, which has occurred during this period. Since the eruption of the primary dentition takes place over the first two and a half years of life it is not surprising that these two factors may sometimes be coincidental. General malaise and discomfort caused by the infection, lower the child's ability to withstand pain so that the sore eruption area easily becomes the focus of attention. However, one has to bear in mind the possibility of local infection in or near the site and this may easily occur where the overlying gum is being crushed between the emerging crown and opposing erupting teeth.

Neglect. In their normal state the gingival tissues are firm and closely adapted to form a streamlined continuum from the crown into the buccal and lingual sulci. Their consistency is tough, firm, can be displaced with considerable difficulty and bleeds only on direct injury. Such a state is maintained in health by resistance to infection, stimulation from food or brushing and freedom from stagnation. Neglect due either to pain from infection or associated carious teeth, or inability, because of mental and physical handicap, gives rise to a simple gingivitis usually reversible if good oral hygiene techniques are introduced.

Characteristics of simple gingivitis are:

Enlarged and swollen gingival margins and papillae.
Halitosis.
Gingival tissues are soft and easily injured and the papillae are like red, shiny, congested swellings between the teeth, easily displaced and bleed freely even on gentle pressure. Significantly, pain is seldom felt unless an acute infection is superimposed on the simple gingival pathology.

Calculus formation in children is much less frequently found than in adults and is rarely seen before six years. It begins where plaque accumulates on the teeth in soft masses at sites where there is stagnation so that it is not uncommon to find it in children who are mentally and physically handicapped. Poor muscular function and lack of detersive foods in the diet give rise to increased plaque formation and poor oral hygiene. An interesting feature of calculus formation is that it seems to occur more readily in mouths with a low caries incidence. Soft adherent plaque accumulates and undergoes calcification chiefly in areas near the orifices of the principal salivary glands, i.e. lingual surfaces of lower incisors and buccal aspects of upper 1st permanent molars. The calculus formation in children is mainly supragingival and occasionally there may be more excessive deposition in diabetic children.

Chronic marginal gingivitis begins when plaque formation is allowed to continue undisturbed. Unless oral hygiene methods are instituted (Chapters 2 and 4), the stagnation which follows encourages calcification to occur in the dense network of cells, cocci, rods and filamentous organisms, so that the inflammatory changes in the underlying gum tissue are perpetuated.

Infection. ACUTE BACTERIAL INFECTION (haemolytic streptococcus). This is not a common oral infection but is sometimes associated with the eruption of teeth, either primary or permanent, and may take place where stagnation, food packing and trauma have caused a localised gingivitis. It may occur with the eruption of 1st and 2nd permanent molars where the condition may progress to a painful pericoronitis requiring urgent treatment. In many cases oral infections appear as an extension of acute infections of the throat or paranasal air sinuses, and may become severe when there is a lowering of tissue resistance.

ACUTE HERPETIC GINGIVOSTOMATITIS (aphthous stomatitis). It is usual to find that this infection, due to herpes virus, affects the two to six year old age-groups and begins with an acute and painful onset. Poorly maintained mouths appear more disposed to it than those that are clean. The sudden onset of the disease is characterised by a bright red gingivitis and the presence in the oral mucosa of translucent vesicles filled with fluid. These rupture to form painful ulcers which vary from 1 to 4 mm in size (Fig. 2.16). They become covered with a characteristic white membrane surrounded by a fiery red margin and are acutely painful especially to salty or acidic foods.

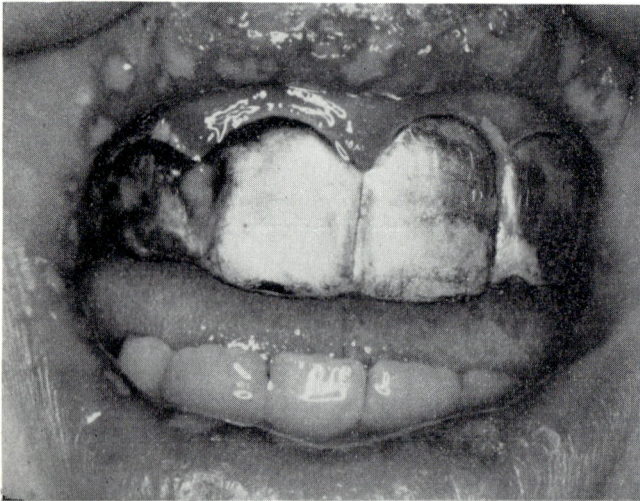

FIG. 2.16. Herpetic ulceration of the lips.

The lesions may occur anywhere in the oral mucosa but very frequently affect lips, gingivae and buccal sulci. Regional lymph nodes become palpable shortly after the onset of the disease, but physically the child has a high temperature, headache, malaise, and severe pain and increased salivation. There is a slight halitosis.

RECURRENT HERPETIC STOMATITIS. Older children and adults are affected by this type of virus infection, which is thought to be carried by over half the population, and becomes manifest when the oral tissues are affected by exposure to trauma, sunlight, and irritants, even in the dental surgery. Emotional stress may also play a part in the recurrence of the disease.

It is characterised by the appearance of painful ulcers similar to those occurring in the acute herpetic infection but more commonly found in the buccal sulci. The duration of the painful stage is about eight days, but the patient is not usually pyrexial or suffering malaise to the same extent as in the acute primary attack. Halitosis is not a common feature.

VINCENT'S INFECTION (acute necrotising gingivostomatitis). It is uncommon in children before the age of fourteen years. The condition is characterised by an acute ulcerative onset which involves the destruction of the crests of the interdental papillae. A pseudomembrane covers the necrotic ulcer in which *Borrelia vincentii* and fusiformis organisms are found. Clinically the affected gingivae are acutely inflamed, painful and bleeding and the necrosis gives rise to a very characteristic halitosis. Pyrexia, malaise and increased salivation are common.

THRUSH (acute monilia infection). The organism *Candida albicans* is nearly always present in the mouth but only gives rise to lesions when there is a decrease in tissue resistance, as in debility. However, the balance of the oral flora may be upset after the use of oral penicillin so that the suppression of some forms of antagonistic organism allows the monilia to increase. In the mouth, the lesions have a characteristic raised appearance in the form of white plaques which are easily detached to reveal a bleeding ulcer beneath (Fig. 2.17).

Drugs. ANTIBIOTICS. Drugs which significantly alter the bacterial flora of the mouth by suppression of particular strains, may allow other, normally harmless, commensal species to assume a dominant role. Such a state of affairs sometimes occurs when the local use of antibiotics in the mouth has continued over a period of time and white patches of thrush become established on the oral mucosa.

PHENYTOIN. Epileptic children receive phenytoin as a part of their therapy (see Chapter 6) but, unfortunately, it gives rise to a

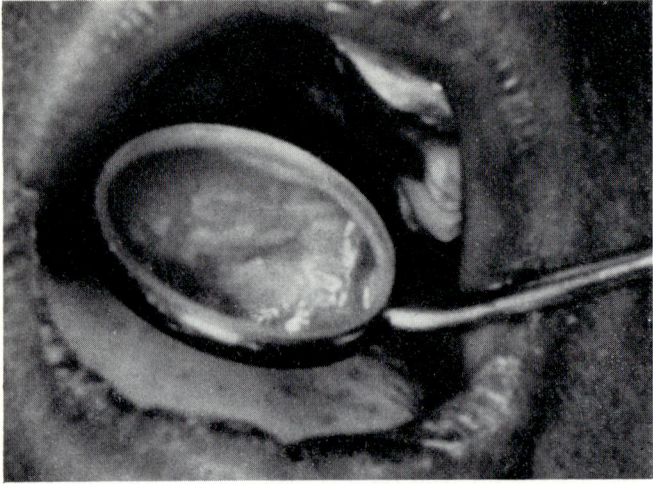

Fig. 2.17. Monilial infection of the palate.

characteristic benign enlargement of the gingival tissues as a result
of an increase in their fibroblast and collagen content (Fig. 2.18).

The amount of enlargment that occurs varies considerably but
may be so extensive as to cover most of the crown tissue in all
segments of the mouth. Although it is not an inflammatory condition,
it more readily occurs and is perpetuated where there is chronic

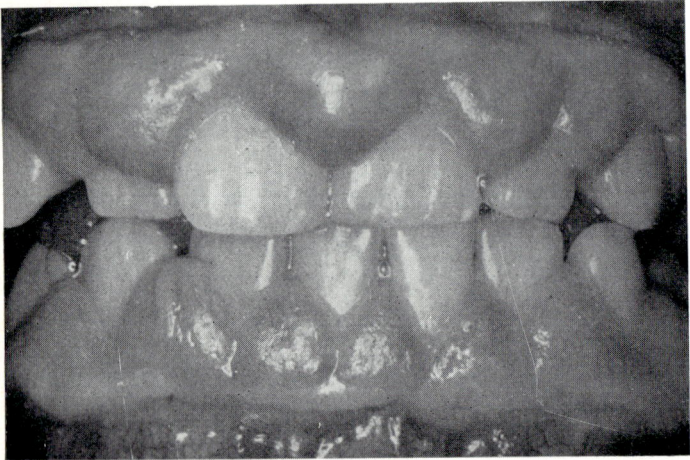

Fig. 2.18. Gingival hyperplasia due to phenytoin (Epanutin)
therapy in epilepsy.

marginal gingivitis and neglect of oral hygiene. It is not associated with a high caries rate and does not give rise to severe periodontal disease.

Trauma. Injury to the oral mucosa frequently occurs as a result of a blow or fall when the teeth and underlying bone may also be damaged (see Chapter 5). Other traumatic injuries, however, may not be so immediate, but as the result of prolonged irritation such as is caused by a poorly designed partial denture, entirely tissue borne, which fits closely into the proximal spaces. The interdental papillae are subjected to prolonged trauma by the stripping effect of the acrylic each time the denture sinks into the soft tissue bed.

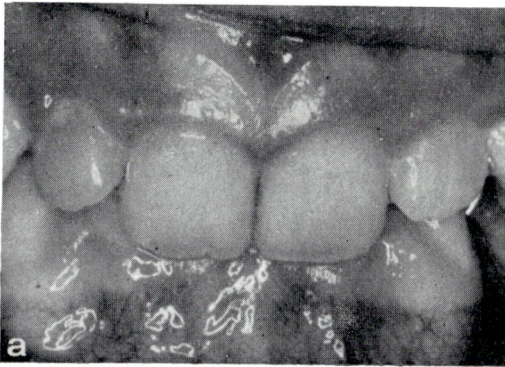

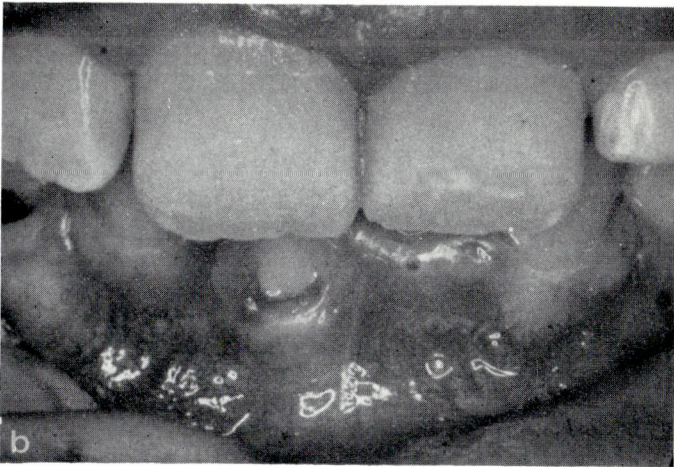

FIG. 2.19*a*. Deep overbit in Class II division 2 incisor relationship.
b. Traumatic injury to lower gum.

Ill-fitting bands and crowns, orthodontic springs and wire arches may also give rise to local soft tissue injury if they are incorrectly positioned or adapted. Where the patient has received a local anaesthetic for treatment, and is inexperienced in its effects, there may be a temptation to chew at lip, tongue or cheek whilst these parts are still insensitive. The resulting ulceration has been described in Chapter 1.

Malocclusion. One of the more worrying aspects of Class II division 2 malocclusion is the increased overbite (Fig. 2.19*a*, *b*) which may bring about a stripping action by the upper incisors, of the mandibular labial gingivae. The condition may be so severe that it may require the readjustment of the incisal angle, irrespective of any aesthetic improvements. The incompetent lip posture associated with Class II division 1 malocclusion (Chapter 7), (Fig. 2.20) allows an unhealthy gingival situation to develop on the labial aspect of 21/12. Hormonal changes associated with puberty may sometimes produce swollen gingival tissues; an effect which fluctuates but is nearly always worse with poor oral hygiene. In Class II division 1,

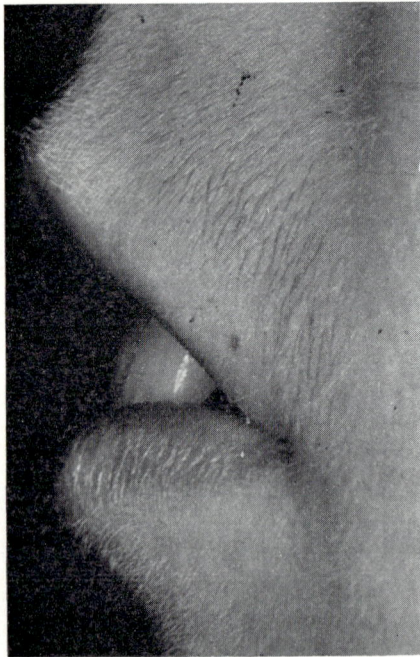

Fig. 2.20. Poor lip posture in Class II division 1 malocclusion.

the poor lip coverage of the labial gingivae allows these to become dry and so encourages bacterial activity which is superimposed on the hormonal changes.

The presence of crowding in the dental arches, expressed in terms of imbrication in buccal and labial segments, has always been considered as a cause of gingival and periodontal changes. Stagnation is certainly commoner in areas where imbrication and calculus formation are more likely.

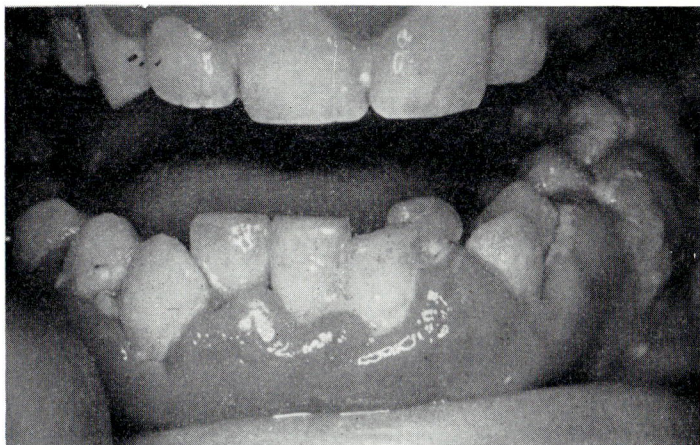

Fig. 2.21. Gingival proliferation and ulceration in a child suffering from myeloid leukaemia.

Underlying pathology. The systemic conditions found in the anaemias and blood dyscrasias are reflected in pallor and lowering of tissue resistance in the mouth. In diabetes mellitus, the principal inflammatory changes are the result of infection superimposed on these factors. There may be additional characteristic changes present, such as the proliferating gingivitis found in chronic myeloid leukaemia (Fig. 2.21), atrophic glossitis present in vitamin B deficiency, and the congested, bleeding gum tissue in the ascorbutic child.

The difficulty in diagnosing these diseases is not where they are fully established, but when the first signs and symptoms are minimal and occur in the mouth. Suspicions should always be aroused when tissue response to treatment is slow or absent and in these cases the child should be referred for appropriate haematological and other tests.

Dental abscess. In the primary dentition, the dental abscess can occasionally occur without painful symptoms, and in the absence of facial swelling it may be discovered accidentally. Because of the relatively superficial position of the roots in alveolar bone, the abscess often points buccally where it rapidly forms a discharging sinus. Perhaps the thin plate of bone which covers the apices is easily destroyed by the inflammatory process so that there is little opportunity for the build-up of a pressure around the roots which constitutes such a painful factor in the abscess of the permanent teeth.

The early release of the intra-bony inflammatory mass into the surrounding soft tissue is shown by the fact that there is little time for the increase in pressure of periapical fluids and the tooth is not pushed out of its socket to the same extent as a permanent tooth. For this reason it is uncommon to find the affected tooth is as painful on chewing as a similar condition in a permanent tooth. However, its periapical disturbance appears to be reflected much more readily by the tooth's increased mobility, an interesting and distinguishing sign when determining the origin of a dental abscess in a heavily carious segment of the mouth.

CHARACTERISTICS OF ABSCESS OF PRIMARY DENTITION. *Pain.* This is not always present but may be severe. It is usually of short duration and as the abscess soon points there is an easing of the pain.

Swelling. Facial swelling, especially of cheeks is very common when associated with primary dentition. May be confused with endemic parotitis (mumps), or associated with submandibular cellulitis.

Halitosis. This is a common feature especially where there is a discharging sinus.

Prior to the development of the swelling, examination of the gum shows an area of intense erythema which is tender to touch. Swellings of the gum are generally superficial and point directly over the apex of the tooth, gathering into a smooth, round sinus. The swelling is often congested and a plum colour and the abscess may point from an interdental papilla causing it to swell and discharge, a feature not usually noted in the permanent dentition. Regional lymph nodes are usually enlarged.

GENERAL SIGNS AND SYMPTOMS. Besides experiencing pain the child may be febrile and show some degree of malaise, restlessness and, occasionally, vomiting.

ABSCESSES OF PERMANENT DENTITION. There is a marked increase in the severity of symptoms associated with abscess formation in the permanent dentition. This may be accounted for by the large root surface, their deep intraosseous position and the relationship of the apices to various muscle and fascial planes and lines of attachments, thus enabling a more profound dissemination of the toxic products. Pulp canals in permanent molars may yield upwards of four times the volume of toxic breakdown products when compared with the primary tooth and, under these circumstances, the child undergoes a greater degree of distress which requires relief either by extraction or drainage. The teeth are painful to the touch or chewing and the affected tooth can be seen to be raised slightly out of its socket and mobile. The associated gum is red and swollen and the patient may have trismus, halitosis and a coated tongue. Regional lymph nodes are enlarged and sometimes painful.

Occasionally the death of a permanent incisor pulp, following trauma or restoration with unlined silicate fillings, may be a painless affair in which there is little evidence of acute abscess formation. Radiographically there is evidence of a radiolucent periapical area and clinically a small sinus is present on the overlying gum without any history of painful swelling. It may be possible to ascribe this lack of reaction to the fact that many of the pulp deaths attributed to the low pH of unlined silicate restorations are, in fact, the result of a small, undetected, traumatic, pulp exposure at the time of cavity preparation. If the pulp remains uninfected, a chronic round-cell infiltration occurs, possibly aided by the low pH of the silicate filling, and the whole pulp cavity gradually becomes filled with degenerating granulation tissue. The disadvantage of this painless chronic condition of permanent incisors is that a considerable area of periapical bone may be lost and replaced by granulation tissue. When the lesion is so extensive, it is unlikely that routine endodontic therapy will resolve the situation unless it is combined with apical root resection (see Chapter 5).

Attrition, abrasion and erosion

These three conditions imply loss of tooth substance by wear and tear and by chemical action.

Attrition. Attrition is very commonly found in the primary dentition where the teeth are softer, but it may be especially severe where the tooth tissue is abnormal such as in cases of enamel hypoplasia and odontogenesis imperfecta. Lack of attrition due to soft sticky non-detersive foods leaves occlusal fissure systems which are deep and stagnating and potentially carious.

Abrasion. Abrasion refers to wear of tooth surfaces produced by chewing against substances or objects placed in the mouth. It is not possible in a great many circumstances to separate attrition from abrasion, except that the latter usually has a more localised distribution. Examples of abrasion are comparatively rare in childhood except for the appearance of the notched incisor edge which results from opening hair grips against the front teeth. Very occasionally children under five years may abrade the cervical margins of $\dfrac{BA/AB}{BA/AB}$ by scratching them with their finger nails. Local irritation may be the cause of this habit.

Erosion. External loss of tooth substances due to chemical action may be closely allied to the problem of the use of comforters. These are used either with a reservoir or are dipped in concentrated, sweetened fruit juices before being placed in the child's mouth (Chapter 3). The low pH of these vitaminised juices combined with their high sugar content brings about a rapid fall of pH on the enamel surface of the upper incisors so that decalcification rapidly occurs with a characteristic distribution. Examples of low pH, sweetened drinks include many concentrated fruit juice varieties and iced lollies all of which contribute extensively to the caries problem.

State of cleanliness

Plaque forms immediately and continuously after the teeth have been cleaned so that there is little hope of ever achieving perfect tooth cleanliness. Plaque organisms produce gingivitis unless their environment is continually disturbed by chewing and oral cleansing. Modern soft, sticky diets have the opposite effect and increase the debris content on the teeth whilst at the same time providing a sugar substrate which the plaque bacteria can quickly transform to acid, forming the basis of the caries attack.

Plaque, with its layered, sponge-like qualities, retains more food debris passing over it than would the polished tooth surface. The significance of this arrangement is that teeth in a poor state of cleanliness will retain more food debris than a clean mouth, which would suggest a good reason for beginning the meal with an apple!

Gingivitis also appears to be more commonly found in mouths which lack cleanliness. Plaque bacteria are responsible for this situation but once the gingivae become swollen and lose their streamlined shape the efficient passage of food will be delayed so that further debris retention occurs.

Enamel hypoplasia, hypocalcification and discoloration

These conditions arise when systemic factors such as temporary nutritional deficiences or the high temperature in exanthematous fevers interfere with the maturation and calcification of enamel. It is characterised by the fact that all the teeth, where matrix formation and calcification are occurring at that time, are affected. Thus the position of the hypoplastic defects will relate the febrile event to the stage of development of each individual tooth. Whilst there is a strong positive correlation between these childhood disturbances and the occurrence of the hypoplasia, careful histories of many children with no exanthematous or nutritional faults may still show these dental defects. On the other hand, some children whose early medical background would make them almost certain candidates for the defects, appear to escape this condition completely. It is impossible in many cases to relate the size of the defect to the severity of the systemic disturbance which caused it.

Mild hypoplasia usually presents as a series of small, discrete pits, with hard bases, almost free from staining and usually with little loss of normal tooth translucency. Another variety exists in which areas of hypocalcification show as stained, mottled enamel, giving the appearance of bands of burnt chalk which are softer than normal crown tissue.

Teeth which are severely hypoplastic show characteristic horizontal bands of deep pits which are usually continuous interproximally and palatally in the incisors (Fig. 2.22). As a result the

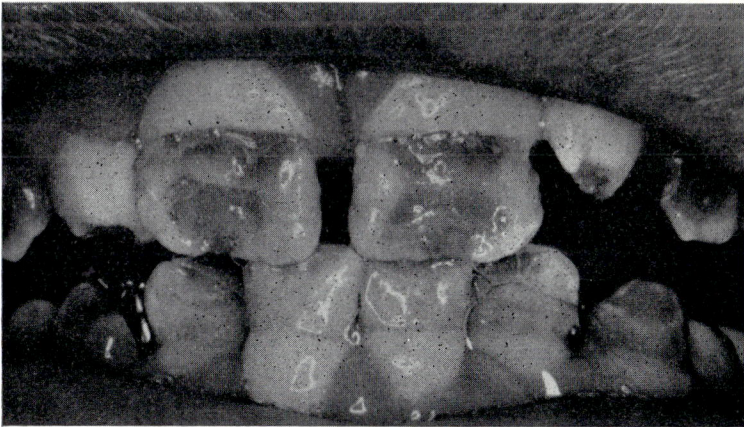

Fig. 2.22. Bands of hypoplastic enamel reflecting a characteristically disturbed pattern of enamel formation.

C

crown may be almost completely divided by a series of horizontal perforations which easily fracture on pressure. There is a considerable degree of staining although caries is not a prominent feature in these cases. Despite the extensive disturbance of the crown structure, the teeth are often very sensitive to thermal changes and to probing.

Enamel hypoplasia in the primary dentition although of little clinical significance in itself may reflect fundamental systemic disturbances during the later stages of foetal life. If this is prolonged one may expect signs of cuspal hypoplasia as the matrix of the 1st permanent molar begins to calcify, and later the permanent incisors will also be involved.

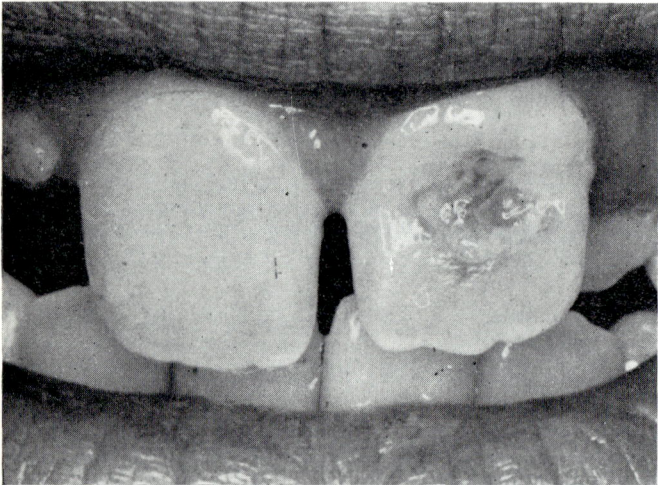

FIG. 2.23. Localised enamel hypoplasia due to earlier injury transmitted through the overlying primary incisor.

Hypoplasia due to trauma and local infection. In this situation individual teeth only are affected and show either a hypoplastic pit or a stained and mottled hypocalcified area (Fig. 2.23) closely associated with the site of injury or infection from the overlying primary tooth. The mechanism by which the defect occurs is thought to depend upon the local destruction of the united enamel epithelium at the particular site, followed by erosion of the enamel by granulation tissue. Injuries to the developing permanent teeth during surgical repair of cleft palate often give rise to hypoplastic defects.

Hypoplasia due to fluoride. One part per million fluoride is accepted as the optimal concentration in the public water supply. If larger amounts are present mottling of the enamel occurs in those teeth developing at the time (Fig. 2.24). Individual variations are large and the clinical appearance of the teeth may vary from a slight opaque discoloration to severe brown mottling. Severe pitting and extensive destruction of the crown may occur in high fluoride areas.

Intrinsic discoloration. PORPHYRIA. In the rare genetic disturbance of porphyria metabolism there is an excessive production of pigment which stains teeth of both primary and permanent dentition a purple-brown colour.

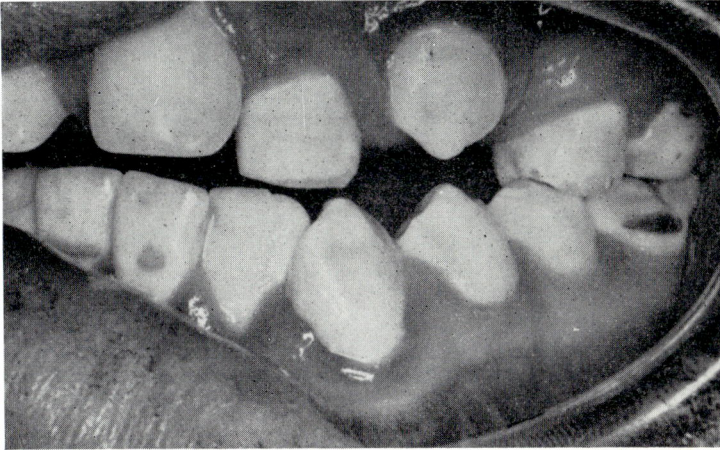

FIG. 2.24. Enamel hypoplasia due to 12 p.p.m. (parts per million) fluoride in the drinking water.

ERYTHROBLASTOSIS FOETALIS. This condition results when the rhesus-negative mother produces an anti-rhesus agglutination as her blood becomes immunised by rhesus-positive foetal red blood corpuscles or sometimes by previous transfusion. The reaction produces excessive destruction of foetal red blood corpuscles and there is characteristic green-blue staining of the primary teeth, but this tends to fade in the incisor area.

DENTINOGENESIS IMPERFECTA. The condition, which is genetically determined, affects primary and permanent teeth which are characteristically a reddish-brown opalescent colour. The enamel of the erupted teeth soon begins to break down and the soft dentition wears rapidly until the teeth are flattened to gum level.

Radiographically, pulp canals are absent or thread-like and the roots are slender and emphasise the bulbous shape of the crowns. Root fractures and unaccountable periapical rarefactions are common. Fortunately the permanent teeth may show only little outward change and the condition may be discovered radiographically by the diminutive pulp canals or when the condition is associated with osteogenesis imperfecta as an expression of a connective tissue disease.

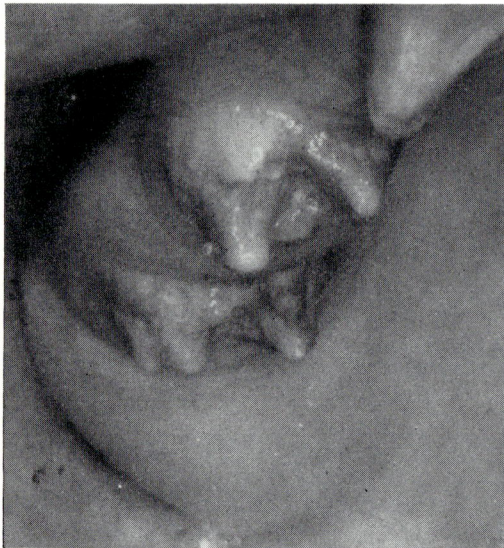

Fig. 2.25. Amelogenesis imperfecta.

AMELOGENESIS IMPERFECTA. This genetically determined condition affects the enamel in both dentitions usually described as either a hypoplastic or a hypocalcific type. In the hypoplastic type, the enamel, although rough and pitted, is hard, and might occur if there had been a partial collapse of the matrix due to a delay in calcification.

The hypocalcific type appears to have formed a relatively normal matrix but calcification is deficient so that the teeth are softer (Fig. 2.25) and easily worn. Brownish discoloration occurs due to increased permeability. It is not uncommon to find that some conditions share characteristics of both amelogenesis and dentinogenesis imperfecta. A feature in these cases is the sensitivity of the teeth to hot and cold stimuli due to excessive wear of crown tissues. Eventually the abrasion may progress so far that the pulp is exposed giving rise to a pulpitis.

Discoloration from necrotic pulp and endodontic therapy.
Pulp congestion may develop following trauma and compression
of periapical vessels. A relatively large volume of stagnant blood is
retained within the crown and rapidly breaks down giving the tooth
a blue or black discoloration. The condition also occurs occasionally
in the primary incisors following trauma. The discoloration is due
essentially to breakdown of red blood corpuscles, the pigments from
which stain the inner walls of the dentine. Whilst this type of discoloration following trauma must always lead one to suspect irreversible pulp damage, it need not necessarily be so. In a few cases the
congestion appears to be overcome and a return to normal pulp
activity follows, although there is evidence of pigmentation from
disrupted red blood corpuscles. Here, however, the discoloration
begins to fade within twenty four hours so that there is appreciable
removal of stain internally, although it is never entirely completed.

There are other situations in which the pulp may die or be
removed without a frank discoloration of the crown. The appearance
of the individual crown itself may not cause comment, but its loss of
translucency makes an obvious difference when compared with
adjacent normal incisors. It is essential to recognise that many of
the traditional drugs used in dentistry, e.g. essential oils, iodine and
especially, silver nitrate cause staining of exposed enamel and dentine surfaces. Their use should, therefore, be carefully restricted.

TETRACYCLINE STAINING. There is a large volume of evidence to
support the highly characteristic tooth-staining effect (Fig. 2.26) of

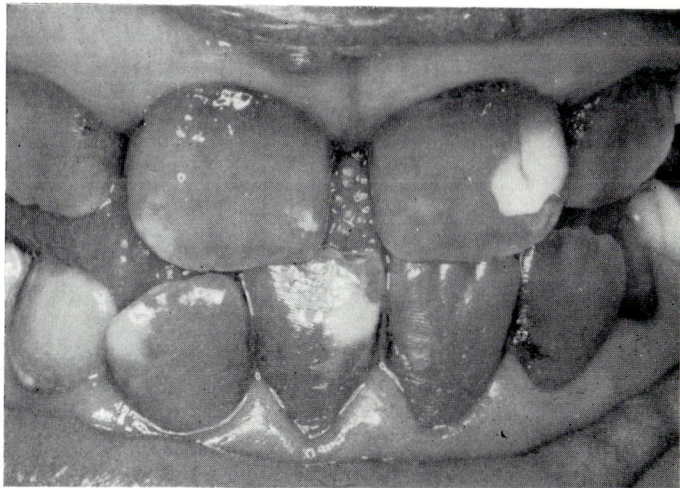

FIG. 2.26. Tetracycline staining.

various types of tetracycline drugs which are now a commonly accepted form of antibiotic therapy. The staining may be from a light yellow to a grey/brown discoloration and may become darker with age. It occurs because the antibiotic is incorporated within the calcifying crown structure. It may occur in the primary teeth where the mother received tetracycline therapy in the final stages of her pregnancy and this was incorporated in the foetal teeth before birth. Subsequently if the child receives tetracyclines between seven months and seven years, this will result in some degree of discoloration of the permanent incisors and, of course, other tooth tissue calcifying during this period.

Hypoplastic enamel defects are sometimes found associated with tetracycline staining, but it is probable that in most cases these are the result of systemic disturbances resulting from the infection for which the antibiotic was given.

Extrinsic discoloration. GREEN STAINS. These are associated with the staining of the remnants of Nasmyth's membrane by chromogenic bacteria. The stain is unsightly and causes anxiety to the parent who may associate it with dental caries. It has a characteristic distribution on areas of the tooth that are newly erupted and little abraded, e.g. at the cervical third of the incisor. The stain can be removed by pumice but will return if the membrane is left intact. Black and brown stains may also occur but do not appear to be of any significance.

Common developmental abnormalities

Over 10 per cent of permanent incisors have developmental abnormalities. The significance of these conditions becomes much more evident under circumstances where the following are affected:

Appearance as in geminated incisors.
Crowding due to increased width of individual teeth.
Interference with occlusion from additional cusps (Fig. 2.27).
Risk of pulp infection as is common in teeth with invaginated crowns.
Spacing in upper labial segment due to diminutive crown forms.

Common forms are mentioned below:

DENS INVAGINATUS. The mildest form consists of a palatal pit at the bottom of which is an enamel-lined short blind tube lying in close relation to the pulp. Caries may lead to pulpitis via this passage and it is not uncommon to find that the patient reports with a dental abscess on an incisor with no history of trauma or obvious caries.

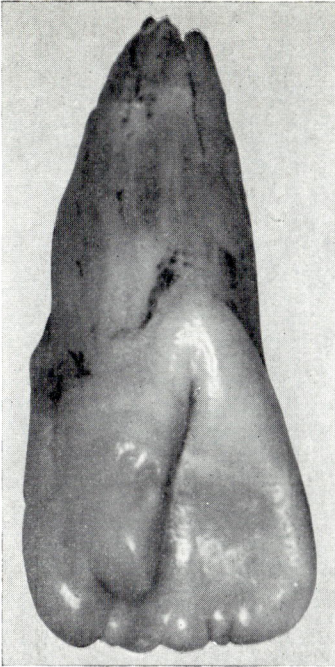

FIG. 2.27. Palatal view of an extracted permanent central incisor with additional cusps and increased crown width.

In the severer forms of dens invaginatus there is an inversion of the hard tissues of the crown, the central part of which may be greatly dilated (Fig. 2.28). Radiographic evidence shows a large centrally dilated space lined with enamel and connected to the surface by an enamel-lined tube. The coronal pulp may be separated into sheets or filaments and is intimately connected with the abnormal internal structures of the crown.

DILACERATED INCISORS. Trauma transmitted to the partly formed unerupted permanent incisor by a blow on the overlying primary predecessor deflects the calcified part of the tooth from its original position. The root portion, still uncalcified, is not deflected and may eventually calcify in its original position out of alignment with the displaced part of the tooth. The situation results in a tooth which either fails to erupt or erupts in an abnormal position dictated by its abnormal root shape.

PEG-SHAPED LATERAL INCISORS. These may occur singly or bilaterally in the upper arch. When they are present unilaterally the other corresponding lateral incisor may be absent. Abnormal and diminutive incisor crown-forms are often found in cleft lip and palate cases.

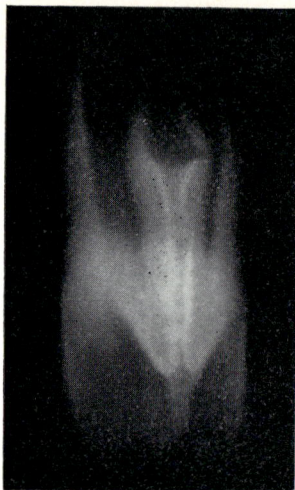

FIG. 2.28. Dens invaginatus. A radiograph of a central incisor specimen showing a well-marked palatal invagination. The enamel-lined tube which is filled with debris leads to a central dilation of root and connects with the pulp.

GEMINATED INCISORS. Crown invaginations frequently occur at junctional areas situated between normal crowns and additional cusp structures and they may represent an unsuccessful axial dichotomy. The more successful this process, the more nearly the crown appears to be divided to such an extent that the attachment of the parts may be by root only. One common feature, however, is the increased width of the crown space which can be restored using a partial upper denture. Where there is a degree of crowding in the upper arch, the remaining upper incisors may be approximated, using a fixed appliance to accomplish root movement.

SUPERNUMERARY AND SUPPLEMENTAL INCISORS. Supernumerary incisor teeth have been mentioned under a previous heading and can, of course, lead to non-eruption of the teeth of the permanent series (Fig. 2.29). However, on other occasions these teeth erupt either palatally, buccally or in arch line. When they erupt palatally or buccally they should be removed leaving the teeth of the normal series. However, when they are in arch line they cause severe disturbance to the teeth of the normal series and following their removal orthodontic treatment will be required to align the remaining teeth.

Supplemental teeth often of the same shape and size as teeth of the normal series usually appear in the incisor area (Fig. 2.30) in both the upper and lower arch. It is important, before deciding upon which tooth to extract, to have an adequate periapical radiograph so that one may be informed regarding the root and pulp form of the teeth in question. Frequently one of the teeth, especially in the

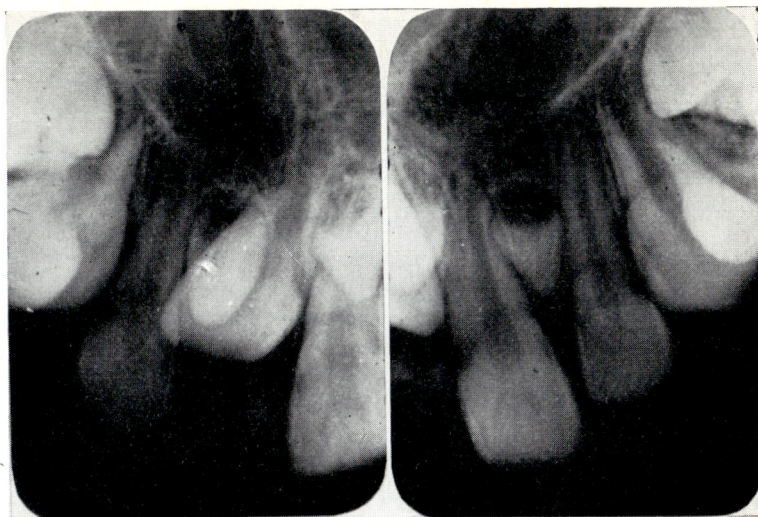

FIG. 2.29. Radiograph of supernumerary teeth in the upper
incisor area.

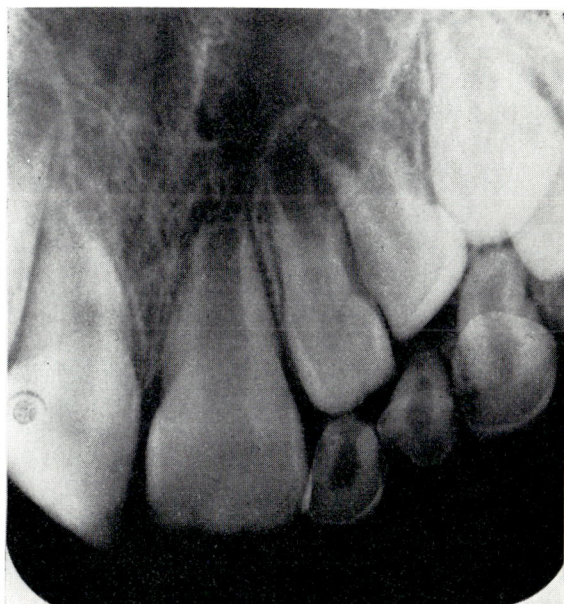

FIG. 2.30. Radiograph of supplemental upper lateral incisors in both
primary and permanent dentitions.

upper arch, is rotated and in these cases, providing both teeth are of equal quality, the rotated tooth should be removed. In the lower arch, when the lateral incisor area is involved, the position of the lower canine should be ascertained before considering removal of the supplemental tooth, to ensure that the canine will erupt and approximate to the incisor teeth that remain standing. Very little in the way of orthodontic treatment is required in these cases.

Impacted teeth. Teeth which are commonly impacted are upper and lower 2nd premolars, lower 3rd molars and upper canines. Factors responsible may be premature loss of deciduous teeth especially where there is potential arch crowding. Unfavourable tooth-tissue ratio and lack of bone growth, both laterally and anteroposteriorly, may result in the exclusion of teeth from the arch.

Delayed eruption due to interference by supernumerary or supplemental teeth may upset the sequence of eruption so that teeth of normal series are diverted from their scheduled positions.

Occasionally the crypts develop in abnormal positions, so that even with a favourable environment within the arch they are still unable to achieve an acceptable position. Such a situation occasionally occurs with $\underline{3/3}$ also in the $\overline{32/23}$ area. The fate of such teeth and their influence on other units in the arch need careful consideration and factors relevant to their treatment are considered below. However, misplaced teeth may pursue aberrant paths (Fig. 2.31) of eruption so that their crowns impact and resorb adjacent roots. Very occasionally, pathological changes occur in the crypts of impacted teeth giving rise to expanding dentigerous cysts.

It is often necessary to make an assessment of impacted $\underline{3/3}$ and to evaluate treatment in terms of the following possibilities:

> *Removal*
> *Alignment in arch after surgical exposure*
> *Transplantation*
> *Acceptance of position subject to annual observation*

Initially the area should be palpated both palatally and labially to assess the position of the upper canines. Radiographs required are periapical views to show root form, bone pattern and intimate relation to adjacent teeth. A vertex occlusal view is useful in order to indicate the relationship of the misplaced teeth to the dental arch and a P.A. (postero-anterior) skull view may help to show the inclination of the teeth to the median plane. The lateral skull view will show the height of the impacted teeth relative to the dental arch and also their angulation in the sagittal plane.

INDICATION FOR REMOVAL OF CANINE. The upper canine should be removed if the 1st premolar and lateral incisor are in contact and the 1st premolar is in good position, without rotation and with a buccal cusp which simulates the canine. This applies equally in the lower arch. When the canine is resorbing roots of an anterior tooth or teeth, and these have to be lost, transplantation of the canine may be indicated, although removal is the most likely course as a prosthesis is eventually indicated. When the mouth is in a poor

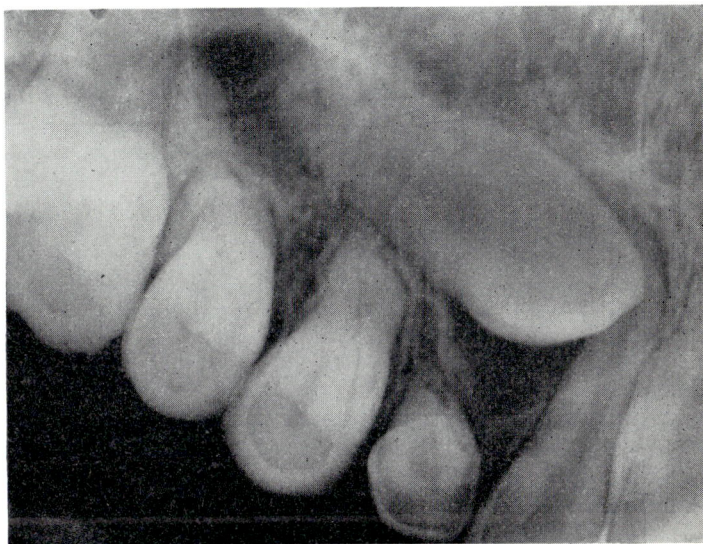

FIG. 2.31. Radiograph of impacted upper permanent canine.

state as a result of dental caries or poor gingival condition, lengthy orthodontic or complex surgical treatment is contraindicated. When the root of the upper canine is curved or extensively bent due to dilaceration, its movement into the arch is very difficult. Even though its removal might be possible without recourse to sectioning of the tooth, transplantation in the appropriate phase is usually impossible because of the abnormal root shape.

INDICATION FOR SURGICAL EXPOSURE AND ALIGNMENT. Surgical exposure should be considered when radiographs show good crown- and root-form and sufficient space in the arch for the canine. An alternative situation is when loss of a heavily restored or carious tooth would provide space for the canine, the root of which should lie in the arch line with the crown displaced palatally or buccally.

The apex should lie no further distally than between the 1st and 2nd premolar roots. With a root position favourable and the crown mesially placed, alignment may be achieved by use of pins or direct fixation of wire to crown by means of polycarbonate cement. Sometimes snaring the crown with wire will provide the necessary purchase on the tooth, but otherwise the use of conventional removable or fixed appliances will suffice to align the canines.

INDICATION FOR TRANSPLANTATION. When the aberrant upper canine is unlikely to respond to alignment with appliances, and would otherwise be removed or kept under observation, and yet space exists for the tooth within the arch, the possibility of transplantation should be considered. When the deciduous canine is retained, its extraction can be used as the basis for 'socket' construction. The presence of a hypoplastic premolar or a diminutive or hypoplastic lateral incisor may be situations which would benefit by transplantation of the misplaced canine.

INDICATION FOR OBSERVATION ONLY. Where the canine lies near the nasal floor, not related to roots of teeth, and without space in the arch to allow transplantation, it is advisable to review it radiographically at twelve-monthly intervals in case the tooth moves and threatens to resorb roots of standing teeth.

Lower canines. When misplacement occurs, it is usually gross, with the tooth lying in the buccal sulcus toward the midline. Occasionally, the canine may be lying across the arch with the crown buccally placed and the root in a lingual position. Removal or transplant can be considered, depending on the degree of arch crowding or spacing, and the need for appliance therapy in general. Lower canines with crowns lingually placed may be treated with appliances, as uprighting when the root is in the arch line is possible.

Transposition. The teeth most commonly transposed are the lateral incisor and canine. In the upper arch the canine may be found erupting between the upper lateral and central incisor and repositioning involves moving the lateral incisor palatally and the canine buccally to resolve the condition. This can be a tedious and hazardous procedure, and the more satisfactory treatment is often to extract the lateral incisor and allow the canine forward in order to complete the arch. In cases where the canine and lateral incisor are completely transposed, the upper lateral incisor is found occluding with a lower premolar or canine, and this is not satisfactory from a periodontal point of view. There is also the problem of the upper canine occluding with a lower lateral incisor. This disturbs the appearance of the anterior teeth as the upper canines can never assume correct arch line due to the contact of their cingula on the lower anterior teeth. In the lower arch the lower incisors frequently erupt with a very distal inclination and the canines erupt buccally close to the central incisors. It is difficult to reposition the teeth in this condition and often preferable to extract lateral incisors.

Assessment of jaw movements

Mandibular movement occurs mainly during speech and mastication, although idle movements are commonly seen. The pattern of the movement is governed by the muscles of mastication, the form of the temporomandibular joint articulation, and occlusion of the teeth. The occlusion has the opportunity to adjust to the mandibular movement during the phase of tooth eruption and later by wear on the cusps. However, the occlusion may disturb the pattern of the mandibular movement when initial contact of upper and lower teeth occurs before the mandible has reached the final phase of closure and whilst it is within the inter-occlusal clearance.

The following scheme should be adopted when examining the patient's mandibular movements. The patient should be sitting upright and as comfortably as possible since this encourages centric relation. The right hand should guide the mandible from the endogenous postural position into occlusion. Providing that the factors governing mandibular movement are in harmony, the mandible will remain in centric relation and reach centric occlusion.

Factors affecting mandibular closure are:

1. *Skeletal asymmetry*. When the jaw opens, it deviates to the side on which the mandible is relatively smaller. This may have occurred as one side of the mandible became larger than the other during the growth phase of the body, the ramus or the mandibular condyle. Conversely, growth on one side may have been retarded. Mild degrees of this condition are more common than gross irregularities. Secondary irregularities of maxillary growth may also be seen. Condylar hyperplasia may be assessed by palpation or a radiograph.

2. *Malocclusion* is normally the commonest cause for disturbance of the path of mandibular closure. The muscles of mastication bring the mandibular teeth to occlusion with the maxillary teeth. Individual teeth, or groups of teeth may obstruct the final phase of mandibular closure, either before or after the limit of the interocclusal clearance has been reached. When the obstruction occurs before this limit is reached, the tooth contact is called a premature contact and the tooth becomes loosened from its supporting structures.

Under the influence of muscles of mastication it moves out of the premature contact position so that centric occlusion may be acheived. When the teeth contact within the inter-occlusal clearance this is known as an initial contact, and the tooth surfaces guide the mandibular and maxillary teeth into occlusion which is not centric and therefore may lead to stress and disturbance in the temporo-mandibular joint. Pain is a common clinical symptom of this condition. The initial contact leads to a crossbite between teeth or groups of teeth and is sometimes seen with upper central or lateral incisors during eruption of permanent teeth, or in the buccal segments where a unilateral crossbite develops between molars or premolars when they are in initial contact.

3. *Muscle spasm* may cause deviation from the normal closure path and is usually caused by infection in the area of the muscles of mastication.

To determine initial contact:

1. Seat patient in an upright relaxed position so as to encourage a centric jaw relation.

2. Move the mandible with the right hand so that the teeth come into occlusion, noting those which are first to contact, and the deviation away from centric relation. The deviation will occur in either a forward or lateral direction, or a combination of those.

When a forward movement occurs, it will lead to an apparent reduction of overjet, but when the initial contact is eliminated during treatment this will increase the overjet, which must be allowed for in the overall treatment plan.

Abnormal mandibular posture. The endogenous postural position is a centric relation of the mandible, but sometimes after treatment of Class II division 2 incisor relationships and occasionally in Class II division 1 incisor relationships, using functional appliances, the mandible may be found to be postured forwards during speech and idle movements. When, however, centric occlusion is reached, a distal movement of the mandible occurs, once erroneously thought to be a distal displacement. This forward posturing of the mandible must be recognised in order to appreciate the implications of treating the malocclusion. The forward posture of the mandible can also be seen on lateral skull radiographs and must be recognised before these films are read.

Assessment of incisor relationships

The relation of upper and lower incisors to each other is easily determined. However, the difficulty of treating the condition may not be apparent unless the angulation of the teeth to the dental bases is noted. In the case of Class II division 1 incisor relationship if the overjet is due to anteroposterior dental base discrepancy and not proclination of upper incisor teeth, tipping the upper labial segment palatally will result in a poor appearance and the teeth will also be prone to relapse. Bodily movement of teeth is required in this condition involving the use of fixed appliances in order to achieve root torque.

In Class III incisor relationship, when the lower labial segment is retroclined and crowding is not present, there is no point in extracting teeth with the aim of retracting the lower labial segment. Similarly, when the upper labial segment is proclined with a reverse overjet, it is of doubtful value to procline the upper labial segment

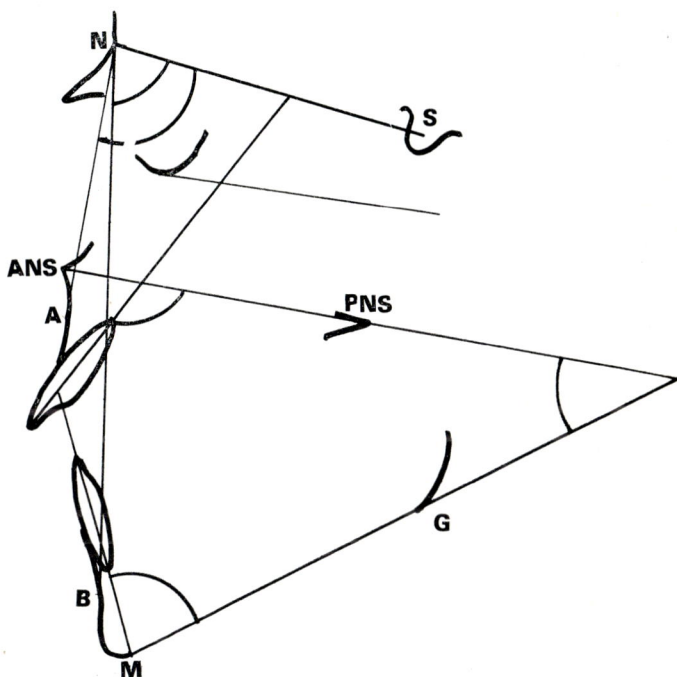

FIG. 2.32. Diagram illustrating the planes used in making a Down's dental-base assessment. Cephalometric points

Key: N = Nasion   B = B point
      S = Sella   M = Menton
      ANS = Anterior nasal spine   G = Gonion
      PNS = Posterior nasal spine   Gn = Gnathion
      A = A point.

further as relapse is likely. The relationship of the incisors may be assessed conveniently by the degree of overjet and overbite and the angulation of the upper and lower incisor teeth to the maxillary and mandibular planes respectively (Fig. 2.32). The dental base relationship can vary in cases with similar incisor relations (Fig. 2.33*a*, *b*, *c*).

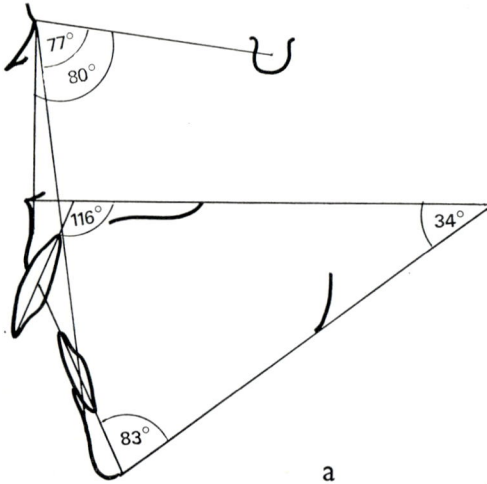

a

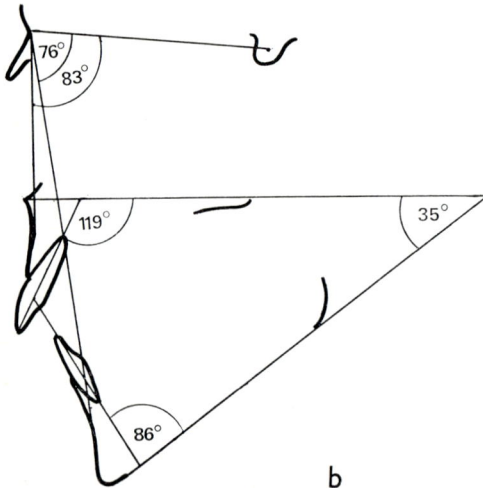

b

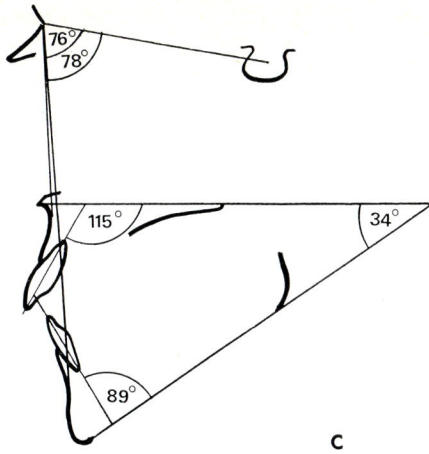

c

Fig. 2.33. Diagrams of Down's analysis in cases of Class II division
1 incisal relationships with the following dental base relationships:
(*a*) Class I.
(*b*) Class II.
(*c*) Class III.

Class I. There is an average overjet of 2–3 mm. The overbite
may be increased, decreased or incomplete (Fig. 2.34).

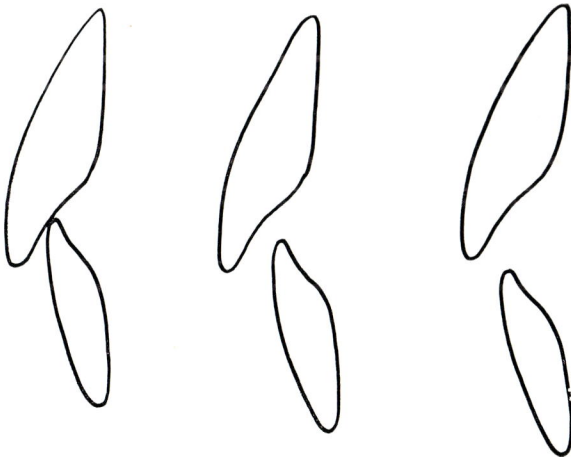

Fig. 2.34. Diagram illustrating variations in overbite in Class I
incisor relationships.

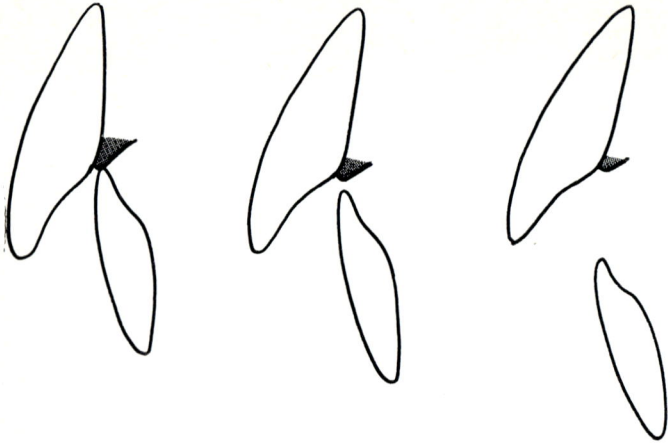

FIG. 2.35. Diagram illustrating increased overjet and varying
overbite in Class II division 1 malocclusion.

Class II division 1. There is an increased overjet, that is greater
than 3 mm. The overbite may be increased, decreased, incomplete
or complete (Fig. 2.35).

Class II division 2. The overbite is increased and complete and the
overjet is reduced. The upper labial segment is retroclined relative
to the maxillary plane. The lower labial segment is in an average
or retroclined relation to the mandibular plane. Classically, either
the 2/2 or 3/3, are proclined in relation to the maxillary plane
(Fig. 2.36a, b)

Class III. The overbite is reduced and may be complete or incomplete (Fig. 2.37). The overjet is reduced to less than 2 mm or
may be reversed. An initial contact of the teeth in the labial segments
may result in a mandibular displacing activity during closure in a
forward or lateral direction (see jaw movement section.)
    Anterior open bite may be present in Class III, Class I or Class II
division 1 type incisor relationships (Fig. 2.38).
    The mandibular displacing activity leads to eccentric occlusion
and this must be allowed for when determining a treatment plan.
For example, if following a forward displacement during mandibular
closure, there is an average overjet. When the displacing activity
has been eliminated, the overjet will be increased as the mandible
is now assuming a centric relation with the teeth in occlusion.

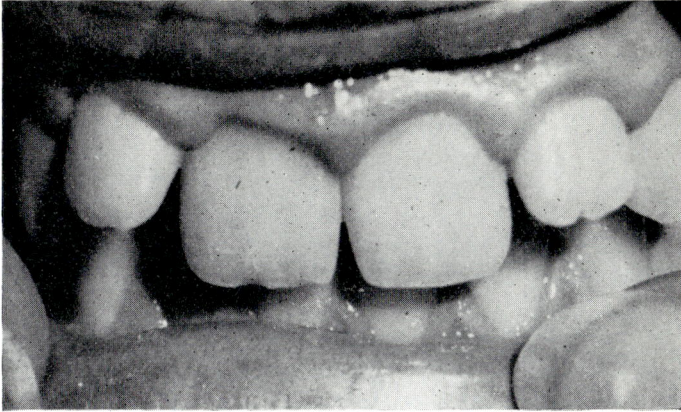

FIG. 2.36a. Proclination of 2/2 in Class II division 2 malocclusion.

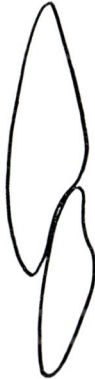

FIG. 2.36b Diagram showing decreased overjet and increased overbite in Class II division 2 incisal relationships.

Centre line of face and upper and lower teeth. Assess the
upper and lower centre lines of the dental arches independently as
to whether they coincide with, or deviate left or right from, the centre
line of the face. This relation may indicate any lateral displacing
activity present and also serves to indicate any drift of the incisor
teeth which has occurred during development of the occlusion.

Assessment of crowding

The relationship between tooth size and size of dental base deter-
mines the degree of crowding and spacing present. Crowding may
prevent individual teeth from attaining alignment within the arch

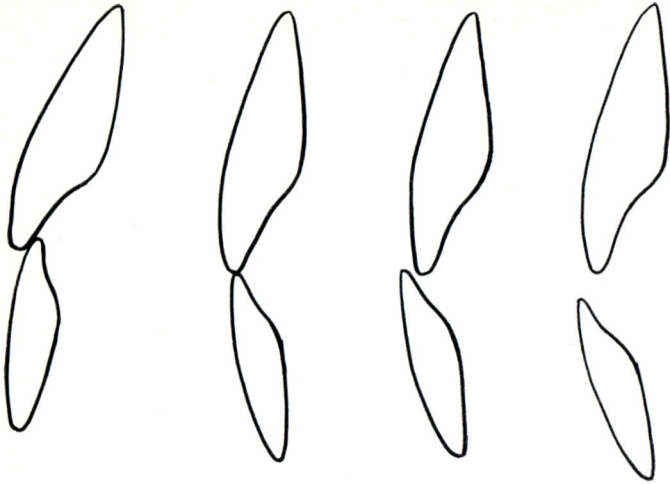

FIG. 2.37. Diagrams illustrating reduced overbite which may be
complete or incomplete in Class III incisor relationship.

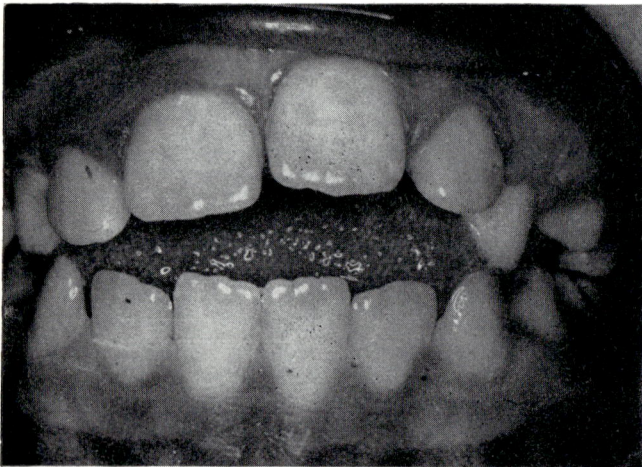

FIG. 2.38. Anterior open bite

or may result in the impaction of teeth. The teeth which become impacted are usually the canines, 2nd premolars or 3rd molars as these teeth erupt later than their neighbours. Radiographs should always be used to show the presence of these impacted teeth and their relationship to the adjacent teeth. Proclination of labial segments is usually a symptom of crowding except when spacing is also present.

Crowding of the upper and lower labial segment in the mixed dentition should be carefully considered, as it may resolve during lateral growth up to eight years old. Loss of deciduous teeth to relieve this crowding by extracting $\dfrac{c/c}{c/c}$ should be bilateral rather than unilateral so as to avoid movement of the centre line. When there is delayed shedding of deciduous molars, and crowding in the premolar or canine areas, it is necessary to bear in mind that 2nd deciduous molars are larger than the 2nd premolars, and also that further growth will occur, so that removal of the 1st premolar only results later in the 1st premolar space remaining intact.

In making the assessment before extracting teeth, it is essential to be certain that the correct radiographic views are obtained so that all permanent teeth present are seen in their developmental positions. This applies to the 3rd molars, which during their prolonged eruption may cause space closure or, where no space exists, imbrication of a previously well-aligned arch.

To ASSESS DEGREE OF CROWDING. It is advisable to follow a set pattern of examination and the following outline has proved to be of value.

Firstly, mentally reposition the teeth in the labial segments so that their angulation to the dental base plane is average, i.e. 109° plus or minus 2° for the upper incisors to the maxillary plane, and 92·5° plus or minus 2° for the lower incisors to the mandibular plane. In order to accomplish this mental exercise the long axis of the incisor teeth and the line of base planes must be drawn mentally on the patient's face and here, of course, an experience of tracing lateral skull films is of value.

Secondly, assess the relationship of the buccal segments to the labial segments, accepting that the canine is the first tooth in the buccal segment. Three possibilities now exist: (1) the canine may contact the lateral incisor, (2) the canine may be spaced from the lateral incisor, (3) the canine may overlap the lateral incisor. In combination with a labial segment of average inclination to the base plane, only in the last category is crowding present if all the teeth are in arch line. When the labial segment is proclined relative to the base plane, crowding will be present if categories 1 and 3 apply and also depending on the degree of crowding where the condition falls into category 2. The foregoing applies where impaction or irregularity occurs in incisal or buccal segment, as this is a symptom of crowding. Where the labial segment is retroclined in relation to its base plane, spacing from the buccal segment is rare unless teeth are absent from the series. The overlap of the labial segments by the buccal segments gives the appearance of crowding, but is not truly the case after the labial segments have been mentally repositioned in to their average relation to the base plane.

Spacing. The affected area of the mouth should be examined with the aid of radiographs for the possibility of partial anodontia. In cases of central diastema this may be due to a midline maxillary fibrous tract or to the presence of supernumerary teeth which can be identified and located on the radiographs.

Assessment of skeletal pattern

Although this is three-dimensional it is usual to make assessments in one plane at a time and then subsequently to view the situation in its entirety. The skeletal pattern may be assessed clinically or cephalometrically. A knowledge of cephalometry is useful when carrying out a clinical assessment (Fig. 2.39).

In order to assess the skeletal pattern one should consider the three main factors:

1. *Antero-posterior variation in position of bone of mandible and maxilla.* This is the dental base relationship. Basal bone is defined as that bone from which the dental alveolus develops. In assessing the antero posterior relationship the points A and B are used for clinical and cephalometric assessment.

2. *Vertical height.* From the above diagrams it will be seen that variations in the maxillary/mandibular plane angle or Frankfort mandibular plane angle produce an alteration in the anterior face height. This in turn influences the degree of overbite present. The labial segments have a certain potential for development which will not be exceeded but may be prevented from being achieved due to soft tissue or skeletal factors.

3. *Lateral variation.* This can best be assessed from models of the mouth or from postero-anterior cephalograms. U-shaped arches are the accepted norm but on occasion the arch may bow out laterally or be contracted to a V-shaped pattern.

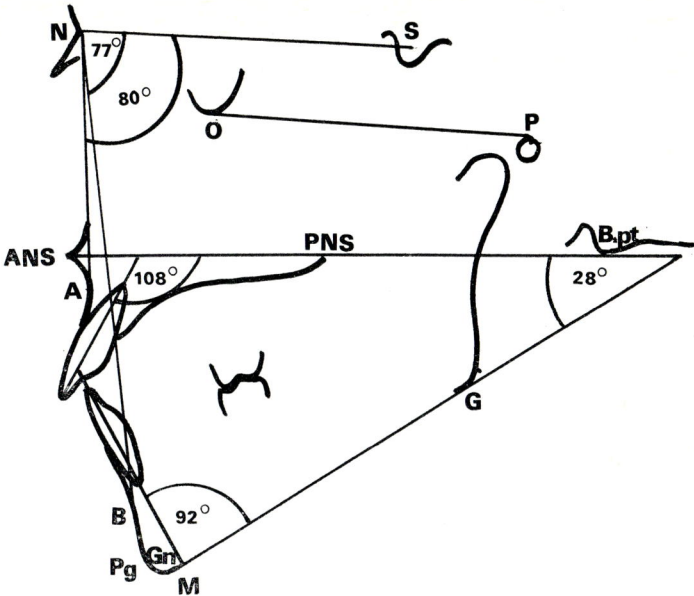

FIG. 2.39. Cephalometric points and average plane angles

Cephalometric points

Key. N = Nasion
S = Sella
ANS = Anterior nasal spine
PNS = Posterior nasal spine
A = A point
B = B point
M = Menton

G = Gonion
Gn = Gnathion
Pg = Pogonion
O = Orbitale
P = Porion
B.pt = Bolton point

To assess the dental base relationship clinically, accept that the upper labial segment is in average relationship to the Frankfurt plane* at 109° and that the average maxillary/mandibular plane angle is 28°. The average inclination of the lower labial segment relative to the mandibular plane is 92·5°. Examine the patient from the side and mentally outline the Frankfurt plane on the ala-tragal line and the mandibular plane as represented by the lower border of the mandible. Now reposition the labial segments correcting the upper labial segment and lower labial segment, bearing in mind that the maxillary/mandibular plane angle and lower labial segment angulation to mandibular plane, are inversely related. The degree

* The Frankfurt plane is a line joining orbitale to porion.

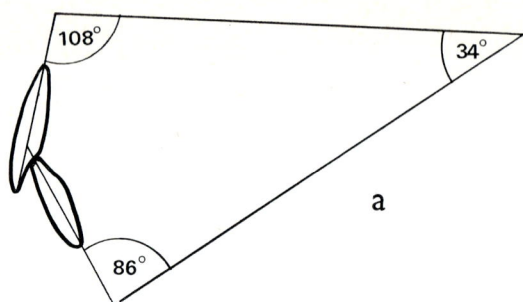

FIG. 2.40*a*. Conversion tracings (after Ballard's technique, 1948) of
the cases appearing in Fig, 2.33.
(*a*) Diagram illustrating Class II division 1 incisal relationship
with a Class I dental base Fig. 2.33*a* after conversion tracing.

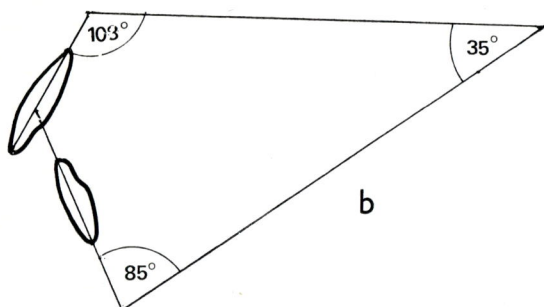

FIG. 2.40*b*. Diagram illustrating Class II division 1 incisal relationship with a Class II dental base Fig. 2.33*b* after conversion tracing.

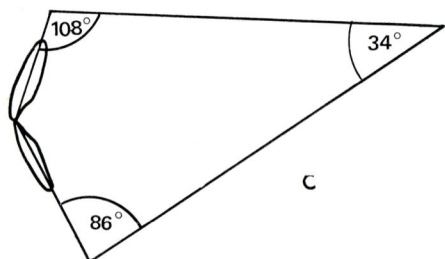

FIG. 2.40*c*. Diagram illustrating Class II division 1 incisor relationship with a Class III dental base Fig. 2.33*c* after conversion tracing.

of overjet present after repositioning the labial segments indicates the dental base relationship (Fig. 2.40 *a*, *b*, *c*).

A second method of assessing dental base relationship uses the relative position of A and B points (see Fig 2.39). To do this the patient is seated in an upright position with the Frankfurt plane horizontal. The operator uses the first finger of the right hand to palpate A point and the second finger palpating B point. When B point is vertically further back by 2 mm relative to A point, a Class I dental base relationship exists. If B point is even further behind than this, the dental base relationship is Class II but if the B point is further forward than A point the dental base relationship is Class III.

One must always be aware of forward posturing of the mandible during clinical and cephalometric assessments as discussed previously. The dental base relationship influences the overjet and the degree of discrepancy is the deciding factor in selecting a method of correcting the incisor relationship. A gross discrepancy in Class II dental base would demand an unacceptable retroclination of upper incisors.

Vertical height of face. The vertical height of the face influences the degree of overbite. The teeth and supporting bone in the upper and lower region have a potential for development which cannot be exceeded. If the vertical height of the face outpaces this potential there will be an anterior open bite. Referring to the soft tissue assessment, it will be essential to recognise that tongue-to-lip activity and sucking habits may interfere with development of the labial segments and produce an anterior open bite. Open bite is thus due to a combination of these factors.

Reduced anterior facial height will occur where there is a reduced maxillary mandibular plane angle. This leads to an increased overbite. The associated soft tissue pattern may result in a lingual inclination of the labial segments so that their growth potential may be fulfilled to produce a Class II division 2 type incisor relationship. In these circumstances trauma of the labial aspect of the lower gingiva occurs and this is sometimes accompanied by a similar palatal situation in the upper arch. It must be recognised that variations of facial height, maxillary/mandibular plane angle and soft tissue pattern produce infinite variation of overbite, the treatment of which is considered in a later chapter.

Lateral variation. This is, in its mildest form, seen clinically as a unilateral crossbite in the buccal segments. It may be due in fact, to an initial contact with accompanying displacing activity of the mandible laterally, during closure.

The maxillary arch may be V-shaped and the mandibular arch U-shaped, allowing an incisor relationship of Class I, Class II or Class III type.

The degree of discrepancy may be altered by the inclination of

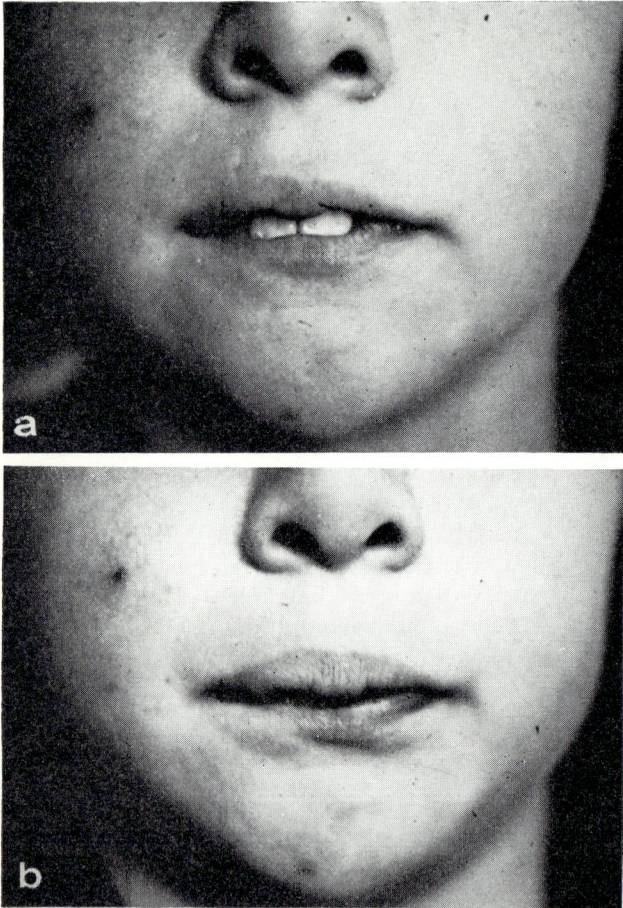

FIG. 2.41*a* and *b*. Incompetent Lips.

(*a*) At rest   (*b*) Lips attempting to form an anterior seal during swallowing.

the buccal teeth on the basal bone. This also applies where the maxillary arch appears to be wide relative to the mandibular arch and may be due to a wide maxillary base or narrow mandibular base, but in the extreme case, the maxillary teeth occlude entirely outside the mandibular teeth. The milder case may be seen with unilateral crossbite and an associated lateral displacing activity during mandibular closure.

Assessment of oral soft tissue morphology

The soft tissues including lips, cheeks, tongue, and sucking habits, are factors which influence the position of the teeth. The lips may be assessed as being incompetent, competent, or potentially competent. Competent lips are those which rest together without there being any conscious effort when the mandible is in its rest position. Incompetent lips are those which are held apart when the mandible is in its endogenous postural position (Fig. 2.41*a*) but may be held habitually together by the patient exerting a conscious effort (Fig. 2.41*b*). There will also be some contraction of the circumoral musculature during swallowing to effect an anterior oral seal. This may be supplemented by contraction of the mentalis muscle. Observation of the patient will show puckering of the skin at the angles of the mouth when the circumoral masculature contracts, and over the chin when the mentalis muscle contracts. Depending on the degree of overjet present, the lower lip may contract beneath the upper incisors or between the labial segments thus aggravating the malocclusion. Lips are termed potentially competent when it is felt that they could rest together when the mandible is in its endogenous postural position, providing that the upper labial segment was repositioned to provide a Class I incisor relationship (Fig. 2.42).

The degree of contraction of the lips and the force exerted on the labial segments during function, influences the position of the labial segments. An expressive behaviour or strap-like action of the lower lip has been described. This is seen during function of the lower lip when it is drawn across the lower incisor teeth in the fashion of a thin red strap and as a consequence their lingual inclination is increased and there is classically a flattening of the lower labial segment.

Tongue. During normal function when the tongue lies within the dental arch during swallowing an anterior oral seal is produced by the lips. However, when swallowing is carried out with the teeth apart the tongue may come forward and seal against the contracting lip and cheek musculature, thus influencing the position of the teeth relative to the dental bases and vertically affecting the degree of overbite.

Tongue thrust. The tongue is thrust forward to contact the

lips during swallowing and if the teeth are apart during swallowing, this will have little or no effect on the occlusion.

When the tongue thrust occurs with the teeth together during swallowing, separation of the labial segments will be produced, ranging from an incomplete overbite to an anterior open bite, depending on the morphology of the hard and soft tissues. Tongue thrust with a tooth-apart swallow may also lead to an incomplete

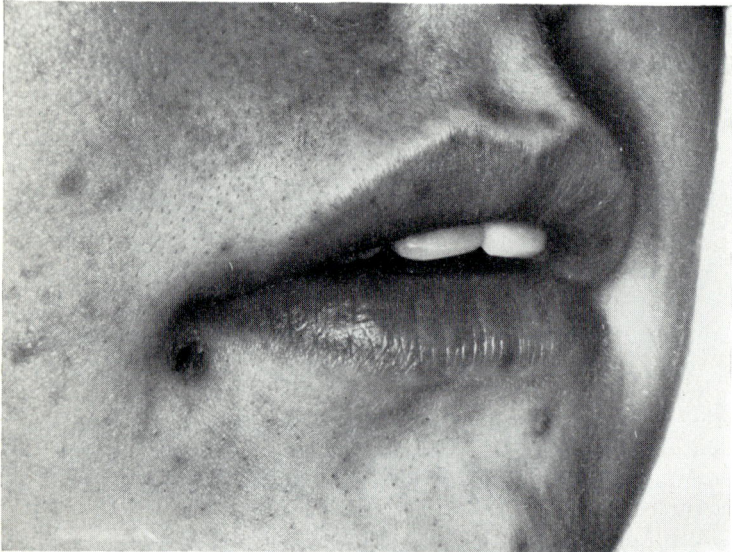

FIG. 2.42. Photograph of a patient with potentially competent lips separated by proclined upper incisors.

overbite being present. The mechanism here is that the tongue moving between the labial segments may lead to proclination of the upper labial segment and also prevent full vertical development of the lower labial segment so maintaining an incomplete overbite. When the overbite is incomplete and the lips incompetent an anterior oral seal may be produced by the lips contracting on the tongue, which rests on the lower labial segment. This may be referred to as a tongue-to-lip resting posture.

Speech irregularities may be associated with these patterns of tongue activity especially, and in particular it has been noted that interdental sigmatism occurs in conjunction with a tongue thrust. In the Class II division 2 type of incisor relationship there is frequently a tooth-apart swallow and in these patients the tongue is held at the back of the mouth during function. The lip line is high and these features combine to allow a bimaxillary retroclination to develop, although 2/2 or 3/3 may escape from the lower lip, to rest on it during function and so may remain proclined relative to their maxillary base plane.

Thumb sucking. Determine during conversation with the patient and parent the intensity of the thumb sucking and assess whether the patient can be dissuaded from further sucking by gentle discussion or whether appliances are required. Examination of the fingers for calloused or soft patches of skin which are exceptionally clean relative to the other hand are indications as to which digits are being used. The callous can be pointed out, together with the deformation of the arch which will be shown by record models. Treatment of this condition is dealt with in a later section.

Tongue thrust and thumb sucking should be considered as habits which can be changed by appliance therapy, and although their presence should be borne in mind during treatment planning they should not present obstacles to successful treatment. The soft tissue pattern should be assessed during the interview but noted down toward the end of the assessment sheet so that the patient need not be conscious of the fact that note is being taken otherwise a false picture may be obtained.

Lip position may be determined easily by observation, but the type of swallow and tongue activity during function demand more experience of the dentist. It is suggested that he engages the patient in trivial conversation so that he may concentrate on observing the soft tissue pattern. It is, of course, important to have the patient in a relaxed atmosphere, seated comfortably and without any distractions in the environment.

Detailed examination of complaint

The operator by following the relevant parts of the assessment to this stage is now in a position to take a closer look at the complaint and to correlate it with the signs and symptoms which brought the patient to the surgery. As a result he should be able to produce a provisional diagnosis.

Provisional diagnosis and special investigations

Additional radiographs may be required to define the exact relationship of dental tissues in a specific situation, e.g. with impacted 3/3; the vitality of adjacent incisors may also be in question.

Similarly, pain on wearing an orthodontic appliance can be due to poor design but may also mask a true allergic response to the dental base material.

Where there is a history of abnormal clotting and bleeding following surgery, further investigation of blood may be required to produce a definite diagnosis.

Case analysis: treatment plan and prognosis

The case analysis is the point in the assessment where the essentials of all the relevant information are assembled. If short cuts are to be avoided and important points missed in collecting data, it is an advantage to use sheets with printed headings or with a multiple answers section where the appropriate remarks can be listed in each case (Fig. 2.43).

Such diagnostic sheets are designed to carry the operator to a logical conclusion with regard to the treatment required and to commit him to an analysis and treatment plan. The analysis is a brief statement of the aetiology and extent of the condition.

Treatment plan. The treatment plan is usually phased into immediate, intermediate and long-term treatment and the way in which these are arranged will depend on many factors such as the urgency of the complaint, e.g. dental abscess, the state of the mouth, the age and cooperation of the patient. In addition to these factors certain other features are of importance when deciding the form of treatment and not the least of these is the expected number of visits, their frequency and also the distance the patient has to travel, particularly if the child is handicapped.

In long term programmes involving continuous appliance therapy the treatment must be planned in such a way that there is regular supervision of oral hygiene especially where stagnation and caries are a problem. Sometimes in the middle of appliance therapy a fall may cause fracture of an incisor and this will inevitably lead to rescheduling the treatment depending upon the progress of the injured tooth. In the event of its loss, the plan of tooth movement will need to be reconsidered.

In forming the treatment plan the dental surgeon should bear in mind the need to involve both parent and child in a long-term programme of dental awareness, but they are only likely to be impressed by these ideals if they find his immediate treatment plans are clear-cut, logical and, above all, practical. The directions which he gives should be specific and built within a framework of a time schedule, adapted perhaps to school or impending medical or surgical treatment.

Prognosis. This is the forecast of the estimate of success for treatment and is based upon experience and case evaluation. The term success is a relative one and for most patients it implies permanent elimination of the complaint.

In the case of children who are severely mentally handicapped excellent conservative work can be carried out under general anaesthesia, but the future of these teeth is often in doubt unless vigorous efforts can be made to improve the oral hygiene. Such examples as these emphasise the fact that the prognosis for a specific condition should always be made against the patient's personality and environment.

FIG. 2.43

Reason for attendance   G.P. treating

Past medical/dental history   Opinion given

Twins   Pathology   Congenital defects   Siblings male/female

DENTAL EXAMINATION

Teeth present——————|—————— Teeth carious ——————|—————

Teeth unerupted ——————|——————   Teeth of doubtful prognosis ——————|————

ORAL HYGIENE
adequate
inadequate

GINGIVAL CONDITION
adequate
inadequate
referred to periodontist

INCISOR CLASSIFICATION
Class 1   Class II div. 1   Class II div. 2   Class III

INCISOR ANGLE
to maxillary plane   average   *to mandibular plane*   average
high   high
low   low

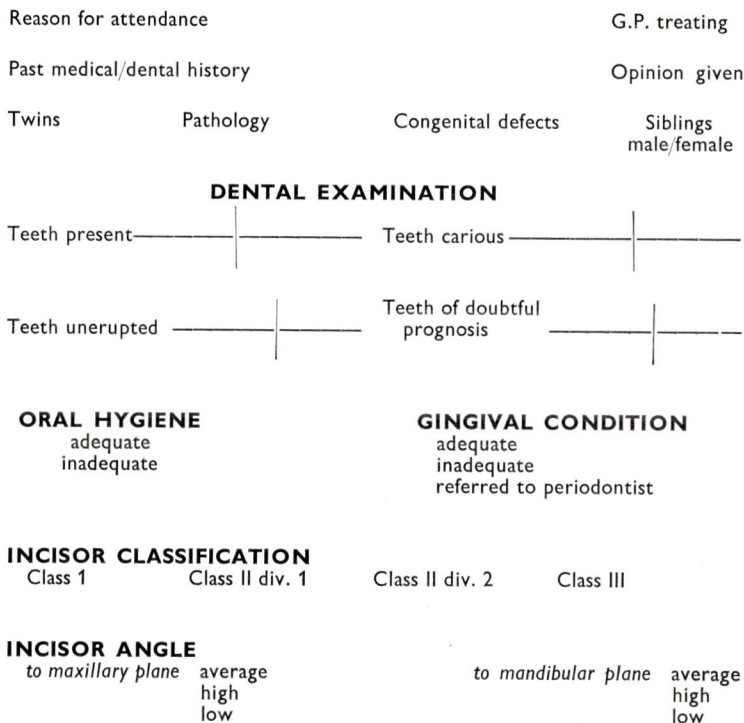

continued overleaf

OCCLUSION

	edge to edge				average	
Overbite	complete			*Overjet*	increase	*Overbite*
	incomplete				decrease	
					reverse	

Anterior		skeletal			left		
	Openbite		*Upper centre*		coincides	*Lower*	centre
Posterior		soft tissue	*line*		right		*line*

Interocclusal Clearance
average
increased   overclosure   traumatic occlusion
decreased

Mandibular displacement during closure
forward
left   *crossbite*   anteriorly
right   posteriorly left/right

Stacking maxilla   *Spacing*   *Infraocclusion*

Molar relation	6 ⎪	I	6
	— ⎪	II	—
	6 ⎪	III	6

Upper left buccal segment *	and *	upper labial segment
Upper right buccal segment *	and *	upper labial segment
Lower left buccal segment *	and *	lower labial segment
Lower right buccal segment *	and *	lower labial segment

SKELETAL PATTERN

		I			average			average
Dental base relation		II	*M.M. angle*		high	*Dental base*		long
		III			low			short

Cleft of lip	left		*Cleft of palate*	primary	secondary
	right			left/right	left/right

Facial asymmetry

SOFT TISSUE PATTERN
Competent lips   Lip to tongue contact
Swallowing—tooth apart   Tongue thrust
            tooth together   Retracting lower lip
Sucking habits   Circum-oral muscle contraction
Speech sigmatism   Mentalis muscle contraction
         dyslalia

* The asterisked spaces refer to the possible combinations of each segment related to the other as described on page 75.

ANALYSIS

	upper arch
Crowding	lower arch
	soft tissue pattern
Adverse	skeletal pattern

CO-OPERATION FACTOR   patient   parent

AIM OF TREATMENT

TREATMENT

1. No treatment upper arch

2. No treatment lower arch

3. Extractions————————————— serial extractions

4. Surgery

5. Appliances
   fixed   a
   removable   b
   class II traction   c
   class III traction   d
   extraoral traction   e

Retention   none
              < 6/12
              > 6/12

Duration of treatment   < 2 years   > 2 years   *Prognosis*   good
                                                                        fair
                                                                        poor

Result of treatment   adequate
                          apical resorption

Fig. 2.43. Printed case analysis sheets.

D

3 The Caries Problem and its Treatment

Dental caries is the result of cumulative chemical injury to the hard tissues of the crown. The restoration of the damaged tissue will in no way prevent recurrence of fresh lesions unless this is accompanied by improvement in the oral environment over a considerable period of time.

The following factors are of practical importance in the caries problem.

Food

Since the Middle Ages the sugar content of the English diet has increased to a level where the annual consumption averages 140 lb per head. It is used either directly as a sweetener for food and drink or as an integral part of sweet and toffee confections. The diet is rich in other sources of carbohydrates, examples of which are confections such as cakes, bread, and especially biscuits containing flour. Modern milling produces a highly refined flour which in the mouth forms a glutinous paste adherent to the teeth. Here it forms a substrate which the bacterial enzyme systems rapidly convert to acid within the plaque.

The Vipeholm Study showed that different types of food vary in the time they take to clear from the mouth and that this clearance rate can be related to the caries-producing potential of the food. In this way it has been possible to grade food substances according to their cariogenic activity and to show that substances such as toffees, because of their tenacious quality and high sugar content are at the top of the list. The persistence of this debris also means that saliva cannot effectively reach the local area beneath the plaque where the fall in pH is occurring and so dilute the forming acid. In the physiological conditions of the mouth, plaque can be regarded as an essential component of caries formation. Its effective removal by oral hygiene techniques would significantly affect the caries rate, but such a task is almost impossible by routinely practised methods. Furthermore success, if once achieved, can only be temporary since the plaque rapidly re-forms and again acts as a sponge and reservoir for the sugar substrate. Even such things as sweetened drinks, and ice lollies, although quickly consumed have long-lasting effects when

their sugary contents are absorbed in the plaque. In experimental
conditions it has been shown that almost immediately after taking
a sugar drink the pH within the plaque falls rapidly below a critical
level at which decalcification occurs. Although the pH falls rapidly,
however, its return to a neutral level is very much slower, in fact
twenty to thirty minutes after taking the sweetened drink (Fig. 3.1).

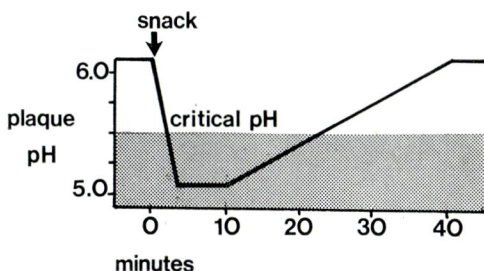

Fig. 3.1. Diagram illustrating the rapid fall in the plaque pH after
the consumption of a refined carbohydrate snack.

From a practical point of view this means that whenever carbohydrate is eaten, its action time in the plaque is much longer than
the time the food is in the mouth, and that this period of activity is
greatly extended where the tooth surfaces are not clean, or where
the refined carbohydrate is very tenacious as in the example of
toffee.

Since the return of the pH to a neutral level is much slower than
its initial fall, the period during which the tooth surface is endangered
is long—irrespective of the amount of carbohydrate consumed at any
one time. If a graph of recurrent sugar snacks is examined (Fig. 3.2)
it can be seen that it is their frequency and not their amount which
produces the most deleterious affect.

If this process is repeated over the whole day, the plaque pH will
be almost continually below the critical level except for a few short
intervals. From these facts it becomes apparent that one 4-oz packet
of sweets eaten economically throughout the day can be almost as
destructive to the teeth as keeping the mouth full of chocolates all
the time.

As bad as this situation is during the daytime, it is worse at night
when the salivation rate is reduced and muscle activity subdued.
During this time there is no benefit from chewing detersive foods
such as apples, and little to disturb the passage of sugar from the
retained food through the plaque to the tooth surface. Most parents
would be horrified at the thought of giving their children sweets in

bed during the night and yet a similar result is being achieved where
a comforter with a reservoir filled with concentrated vitamin syrup
is being used, or where the small child is allowed to go to sleep
sucking his feeding bottle containing sweetened milk food preparations. Sweet foods and drinks are great comforters and are given
liberally to children who cry in the night because of pain or discomfort. Once the habit starts it is difficult to discontinue and the
child's sleeping pattern becomes conditioned by the use of these aids
to sleep.

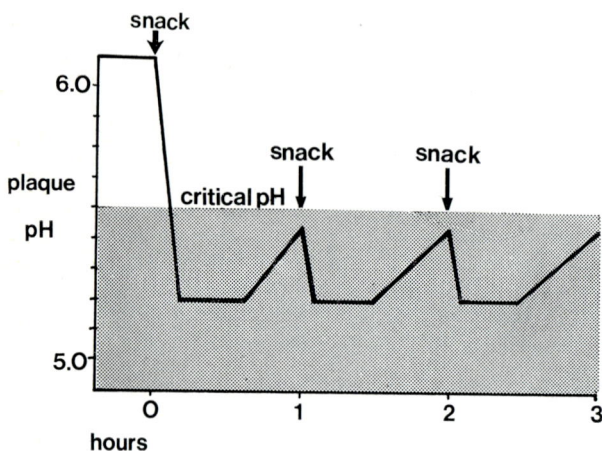

Fig. 3.2. Diagram illustrating the way in which the plaque pH is
kept within a critical destructive range by repeating the carbohydrate
snacks.

Availability. Sweets, biscuits and cakes are relatively cheap,
and available in every public thoroughfare. Their promotion and
pleasurable acceptance, publicised on television and in print, is woven
into the structure of society. When compared with protein, carbohydrate confections have good keeping properties so that they are
the food of choice away from home especially on journeys. They act
as stopgaps for those who miss regular meals and easily become a
habit at tea breaks, at home, school and work. The domestic biscuit
tin is a principal culprit where the young child is involved. He learns
soon where it is kept and how to get to it especially when he does
not fancy his prepared meals. Food which is badly selected and
unattractively prepared, does not automatically become appetising
when it is cooked. Neither do frequent repetitions of any particular
dish improve its gastronomic qualities. Furthermore, cooking is

expensive and time consuming and if the result is unsatisfactory the child is likely to be offered carbohydrate as an alternative.

The social status of women is changing rapidly and many find that they prefer to take up some part-time employment in order to finance a higher standard of living. Others dislike domestic life and many nursery schools take in young children whilst both parents are at work. This state of affairs gives the mother a higher spending ability, some of which is used to provide her child with presents and rewards after a day's absence. There is perhaps an element of over-indulgence to compensate for her voluntary separation from her child whilst at work.

Biscuit factories, confectioner's shops and food markets employ a great number of married women on a full or part-time basis and there are frequently opportunities of cheap carbohydrate 'handouts' to employees who, understandably, over-purchase on these occasions.

A habit factor is often present so that the child may need to suck in order to get off to sleep. This seems to be especially true while the child is teething. If the mother is advised to abandon the feeder at sleep times, the child may find it difficult to sleep and the continuous crying will soon reduce the parent to the state where life becomes intolerable. The child needs to suck for comfort and if it can only derive this from sucking a bottle then he should be allowed to continue but without the harmful contents such as additional sugar or low pH of concentrated fruit juices. Plain water or fresh T.T. milk provide an excellent and acceptable substitute. Continuous crying during the first months of life will require medical advice and it is often found that colic can be relieved by medication with anti-spasmodic agents.

Oral factors

Little is really known concerning the contribution of the various factors such as crowding, occlusion and muscle activity in the clearance of food debris from the mouth, and much of what is taught is traditional rather than factual. Such features as lack of tooth cleanliness and gingivitis are associated with greater debris retention, but this does not mean that high scores for these factors will necessarily lead to a high caries rate.

One of the most disappointing aspects of dental health programming is that routine toothbrushing is not effective in controlling caries although it has advantages in maintaining a healthy gingival condition. If dietary carbohydrate can be indicted as a principal culprit in producing dental caries it would appear likely that thorough brushing immediately after consumption would help to clean some from the teeth and also reduce the number of oral bacteria. However, if one considers that children attending routine dental clinics fall far short of the optimal oral hygiene programme even when under treatment it is not surprising that the result is not effective.

Genetic factors appear to have little influence on dental caries as compared with environmental factors and it is certainly true that children often acquire their oral hygiene and dietary habits from their parents, but blame their caries on their inheritance. Very little is known about the relationship between malocclusion/crowding and dental caries. It is always assumed that crowded mouths with irregular teeth incur a higher debris retention. There seems little evidence to support this clinical impression. In Ancient Egyptian jaws, many showed evidence of dental caries, perhaps surprisingly in a race where there was practically no arch crowding and nearly always extensive attrition.

Preventive Treatment

Diet counselling

Personal consultation gives the ideal opportunity to discuss individual problems, idiosyncrasies and to evaluate specific solutions. Although it requires both time and patience to be effective, it is of especial value in cases where there are major diet faults as in the habitual addition of concentrated fruit juices in a comforter for the very young. To help him in these and similar circumstances the dental surgeon should carry in his mind a comprehensive list of possible dietary sources and practices which may be contributing to the condition.

Extensive investigations of the child's total protein, fat, carbohydrate and vitamin consumption are not necessarily relevant to the caries problem and the dentist should concentrate on the following.

1. **Refined carbohydrate snacks** (*a*) How often does the child have snacks and what form do they take, e.g. sweets, biscuits, fruit drinks, vitamin supplements, and what is the total daily and weekly consumption?

(*b*) When does he receive them, e.g. between meals, in bed, at school? When he has a comforter?

(*c*) What is the source of the sweets, e.g. parents, brothers or sisters, grandparents? School tuckshop or nursery school?

Diet sheets may be of help, but immediate verbal evidence especially from the child is more likely to reflect the true state of affairs. Occasionally, however, the dietary history remains obstinately unrevealing and it may be necessary to recall the routine of a typical day with parent and child before the relevant information comes to light.

In any discussion with the parent and child, the dentist has to bear in mind that caries is the cumulative result of dietary faults. These may not be recent in origin and so it may be necessary to reconsider the problem in terms of caries activity over the previous year. Unless he is prepared to do this he may find he is now collecting information which bears little relation to the real historic cause of the caries problem. It is interesting how few parents or children volunteer information even when they know from previous discussions and experience the nature of the dietary fault. It is a parent's self-defence mechanism which makes her try to transfer any blame to some natural failing in the quality of the teeth, possibly a developmental or prenatal error which no one could have controlled. However, it is no real kindness to allow her to continue in this belief, since it encourages an unsatisfactory dental attitude in that she may feel all treatment is futile because the teeth themselves are faulty.

2. **Detersive qualities of diet.** Modern methods of preparation condition food to such an extent that little chewing is required. This is brought about partly by the highly efficient selective milling process. Precooked and processed foods are common, but natural foods which can be eaten and enjoyed in the raw state, for example, apples and other fresh fruit are a costly item of family expenditure. What is the detersive quality of the diet? It is the rough fibrous consistency in which the particles do not bind together during chewing but form a phase in which they are separated in a salivery medium. Most fruit and vegatables, with some notable exceptions, fall into this category and much more so if they are eaten uncooked. It is the crisp quality of these foods which allows each particle to retain its rigidity for the maximum time whilst the bolus is being formed. Each fragment may then act individually to clean surfaces over which it passes. Such a situation is beneficial for the tooth if carried out regularly, since it not only assists in removing food debris but also ensures that the rapidly forming plaque is frequently disturbed. The acid flavour of fruit adds a further advantage by increasing the salivatory response. Even under such favourable circumstances, however, there are areas deep in the fissures and around the contact points of the crowns where this detersive action will not be effective, and it is for similar reasons that these shadow zones are just as difficult to clean by toothbrushing. It is likely

therefore that plaque removal can never be completely successful in these areas by normal means and they will always constitute an 'at risk' factor in the aetiology of caries. Unfortunately, the tooth morphology also favours food debris retention in these areas so that undisturbed plaque and sticky foods can contribute in a simultaneous and prolonged manner.

Wear of tooth surfaces so characteristic of the Egyptian era, and also in the Iron Age and Saxon times, was due to the inclusion of grit and other abrasive contaminants in the food. Even so, the benefits which resulted in fissure elimination and contact point wear did not ensure complete protection from caries. Modern civilised diet contains few such abrasives, but it is important to recognise that rough, raw foods, remove large amounts of plaque and reduce the associated bacterial flora. Although the layers quickly re-form on the tooth surfaces the generous use of detersive foods will effect a beneficial balance in the level of plaque elimination.

The intrinsic pleasure of the chewing activity in order to extract the full flavour from food is one reason why gum and chewy toffees are such favourites. Oral stimulation is an important part of sense gratification and it is unfortunate that so little in the daily diet contains this exciting quality. Sweetness and tastiness are readily added by means of flavouring agents so that once in the mouth, the full flavours are immediately available without the need for chewing to extract them. Oral gratification begins with breast-feeding and lack of these early experiences, coupled later with a dull soft food may compel the child to seek more rewarding delights in the big taste products of the sweet shop or the biscuit tin. Later, in puberty, smoking may also be linked with the unfilled desire for oral gratification. The qualities of comfort, pleasure and reward, are thoroughly exploited by modern television commercials and press. It is not surprising that under such circumstances it is difficult for patients to follow advice for restrictive diets and particularly so for very young children who can make large emotional demands on their parents in order to obtain sweets. If the environment of the teeth is to become more favourable, substitution in the diet becomes the only practical way to obtain beneficial changes. It means that the child's eating pattern will not be immediately stopped but gradually changed and in order to bring this about effective motivation must be supplied.

The promotion of an idea depends upon supplying it in a form which attracts the individual and in a situation where he can identify himself. It is, for instance, not sufficient to point out that a good home-care programme will give the child sound teeth or, worse still, that she will have to come to the dentist less often! The best motivation is positive and personal in its approach, and may need to be supplied at a level where the boy sees himself climbing out of the lunar module, or she recognises that a camera smile means showing her teeth to the whole world and not just the dentist. Once she has become interested she should be shown the simple dental health steps already described. If the patient has any doubts about the poor state of the oral hygiene then a demonstration can be made using disclosing tablets. Even young children are impressed by the resulting appearance of the teeth and the scheduled prophylaxis which follows gives a sense of a fresh start to their endeavours.

Practical steps for improving pattern of diet

1. The diet pattern and the period when it operates must be determined.

2. The usual sources of biscuits, toffee, sweets and chocolate must be excluded from the home and parents of young children should tactfully inform relatives and friends.

3. There should be no interference with the main meals of the day. The child should be encouraged to eat at these times so that there is less need for snacks between meals.

4. Fresh fruit should be given for mid-morning break at school and money, traditionally provided for biscuits at the tuckshop, can be placed in a child's savings account newly opened for that purpose. Parent-teacher associations can do much, by their criticism, to prohibit the sales of biscuits on and near the school premises.

5. At home the a.m. or p.m. break should substitute an appetising cheese snack, e.g. cheese on toast and for those who prefer it, yoghurt or milk shake instead of biscuits. Fresh fruit should be available.

6. Lapses in diet control must be expected and are often due to poorly prepared meals which are presented in an unattractive manner. The fortuitous arrival of large consignments of chocolates by post and the very occasional indulgences of this type by the whole family are of no significance provided the general daily eating routine is adhered to. However, care should be taken that sweets so obtained are eaten straight away and not hoarded for prolonged gratification.

It becomes evident that the advice given to the parent should be practical and should suggest measures which the dentist would reasonably expect his own children to carry out. It should be flexible in its approach and free from criticism which merely condemns without regenerating the child's confidence in the dental programme.

Advice

1. *It should be fundamental.* Unsupported statements such as 'You must clean your teeth' or 'You must cut out sweets' should be avoided since they are immediately recognised as yesterday's old depressing negative phraseology, by the patient. Instructions such as these make two grave assumptions, namely that the patient knows what is meant by 'sweets', i.e. things that are bad for the teeth and that he also knows the circumstances in which the most injurious effect occurs. The second assumption involves the principles of oral hygiene practice. They are not simply concerned with a ritual brushing but a brushing which is effective both in time and thoroughness and one closely linked with detersive dietary components such as apples, which also help to remove plaque.

2. *The advice must be simple.* So simple, in fact, that both parent and child can understand it. They can be asked to write down these three main rules whilst they are in the surgery:

> When and how to clean the teeth.
> The good things to eat.
> What to do about those snacks, especially when there is an increasing caries rate.

3. *The advice must be practical.* The patient should be told what sort of brush to buy and he must be shown with models the way it is designed to work. It needs a little extra effort, but he should be asked to bring his new brush on the next visit and show how well he is managing. Fones method (Fig. 3.3) is easily learned but electrically powered toothbrushes may be an advantage for handicapped children (see Chapter 6). The technique should always be so simple that the child can easily succeed with it. When this has been achieved he will be encouraged by the praise he receives and the confidence will allow gradual modifications to improve the quality of the method.

What practical help can the patient be given with the diet? The operator should be concerned not with an ideal dietary standard but with what he knows of the practical issues concerned. He must ask himself how successful he expects his patient to be in restricting the consumption of cariogenic foods rather than absolutely prohibiting them.

Operative Treatment
Prophylactic methods

EXTENSION FOR PREVENTION. Although it is impractical to remove fissures for all non-carious 1st permanent molars the idea has considerable merit especially when it is realised the dentist has difficulty in finding any of these teeth unaffected by caries by the time the child is twelve years old. The most valuable measure carried out on carious teeth is the prophylactic extension of the cavity outline to

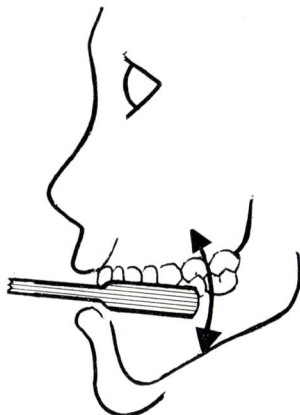

FIG. 3.3 Toothbrushing by Fon method.

include the whole of the coronal fissure system, a technique which should be performed on all affected primary and permanent molars. It is reasonable to assume that the conditions which are unfavourable for one part of the fissure system will affect the rest of it in the course of time.

LOSS OF 1ST PERMANENT MOLARS. Extraction of $\dfrac{6/6}{6/6}$ once suggested as a method useful for reducing the caries rate should not be considered unless the quality of these teeth or the state of crowding is so adverse as to warrant it. Such extractions, in fact, have been shown to have no effect on the subsequent caries rate.

TOPICAL APPLICATION OF FLUORIDE SOLUTION. Fluoride salts may be applied to the teeth in a variety of forms, for example, as a component of toothpaste or as a gel designed to remain in contact with the teeth briefly over a specific period. Whichever form is used, there are usually serious drawbacks in the efficiency of techniques, incompatibility of chemicals and in time consumption. They all stem from the interest in clinical trials in the 1940 and mid-1950 periods, based on the application of either 2 per cent sodium fluoride or 8 per cent stannous fluoride solutions to the teeth. The latter has been estimated as between 20 and 60 per cent more effective than the former. Some of the best results indicate that the caries reduction may be as great as 65 per cent, although a 35 per cent reduction is given more commonly as an optimum figure.

Preparation of the stannous fluoride solution. The stannous fluoride solution is unstable and needs to be freshly prepared for each child. This is accomplished by dissolving 0·80 g stannous fluoride powder in 10 ml distilled water in a plastic container and discarded after use.

Technique for application of stannous solution. When the restorations have been completed, the application of fluoride must be preceded by a thorough prophylaxis using a pumice/glycerine paste and abrasive linen strips applied between the teeth to cleanse the proximal areas. The teeth are isolated with a saliva ejector and cotton rolls and the mouth treated in quadrants. Each is first dried with compressed air and then the fluoride solution applied on cotton-wool applicators by which the teeth are kept moistened during a four-minute period. The other quadrants are treated similarly, but no rinsing, food or drink should be allowed for one hour following the application.

Fissure sealants. Although a number of fissure adhesives are being developed, one currently under review is that supplied by L.B. Caulk Company, Milford, Delaware, U.S.A. It consists of a clear liquid containing principally bisphenol A and glycidyl methacrylate and a methylmethacrylate monomer in which is dissolved 2 per cent benzoin methyl ether. The last constituent acts as an ultra-violet light sensitive catalyst.

Before applying the liquid to the fissures and pits, the teeth must be thoroughly cleansed and their occlusal surfaces dried. They are then conditioned for one minute with a drop of 50 per cent phosphoric acid solution containing 7 per cent dissolved zinc oxide (percentages by weight). The adhesive is applied by brush and hardened in twenty to thirty seconds by exposing it to ultra-violet light focused intraorally on to the tooth surface.

Over a two-year period, caries reductions of 99 per cent in occlusal fissures and pits of permanent teeth and 87 per cent in deciduous teeth have been achieved. Where the fissure adhesives are used on teeth already treated by applications of topical fluoride solutions, they may serve to offer additional protection in the relatively vulnerable occlusal areas.

Restorative techniques for primary teeth

PREPARATION. The young child fatigues more easily and is more restless in the dental chair even if the operative procedures are painless or carried out under local anaesthesia. About 10 per cent of children below the age of seven are amenable to the use of rubber dam, but a much larger percentage are usually so well controlled that other methods of saliva elimination are effective. The use of ultra-high speed airotor cutting techniques is now the normal with cooperative patients and for this the water coolant is essential. Under these circumstances this would seem to reduce the usefulness of rubber dam except when endodontic treatment becomes essential, where it acts as a barrier against contamination and also protects the patient against swallowing reamers.

The use of high-speed cutting instruments carries a risk of mouth injury if the patient moves unexpectedly. It is for this reason that whenever possible an effective local anaesthesia should be established before beginning cavity preparation and that a flanged saliva ejector should be employed to deflect the tongue when working on the lower arch. The mirror head can also act as a protector if placed between bur and soft tissues. Rigid discs, either diamond or carborundum, should never be used in the oral cavity unless they are confined in the appropriate guard.

Important physical features of primary molars (Fig. 3.4)
1. Smaller than first permanent molars in size with bulbous cervical shape. Colour is white.
2. Roots curved to enclose premolar.
3. Pulp horns are slender but extensive and pulp volume is relatively large.
4. Less sensitive and softer to cut.
5. Cervical enamel prisms lie in horizontal plane.

Removal of caries. Cavity outline will be influenced by the position and extent of the caries so that it is of practical importance to remove the bulk of the decay before the preparation is undertaken. Right-angled chisels will quickly remove the unsupported carious enamel and spoon excavation can then clear the bulk of the decayed material.

Occasionally in deep cavities there is an element of doubt when it comes to removing the last remnant of soft dentine for fear of pulp exposure. The operator must consider how far he is justified in leaving such material in the floor of the cavity and inserting a restoration on top of it.

Providing there is no evidence of periapical disease and the tooth has been without symptoms the following principles should guide the operator:

(*a*) The final trimming in the area to the last remnant of softened dentine should be carried out with a large rose-head bur at slow speed, as it offers a more controlled and gradual removal of softened tooth tissue than a hand excavator and is less likely to slice into the pulp. It is the quality of softness of the dentine which decides the

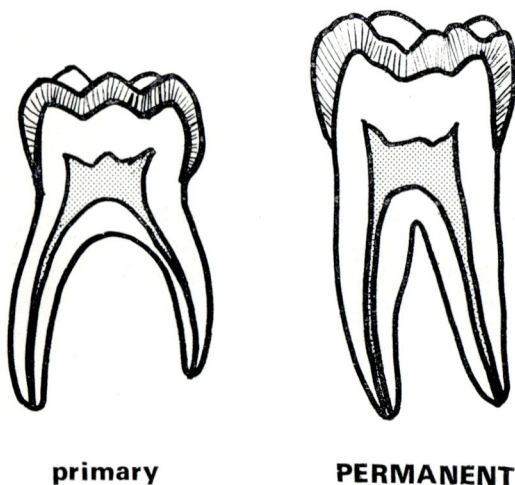

primary   **PERMANENT**

Fig. 3.4. Diagramatic comparison of primary and permanent molars.

operator whether he should continue excavating, but this sensation should be carefully tested with a probe and not the excavator.

(*b*) No chemical application should be made to the soft dentine, since these will not effectively sterilise the tissue but may cause pulp irritation in deep cavities.

(*c*) A layer of calcium hydroxide paste should be placed over the small soft area and, due to the restricted space, no further lining material added in the primary molars, although it will be necessary to add a cement layer in the permanent teeth.

(*d*) It is generally found that there will be no further progress of caries in the cavity floor which becomes hard and supported by a good layer of secondary dentine. However, if caries is left in the wall, especially at the enamel-dentine junction, it will progress.

Cavity preparation. The two parts (*a*) lock and (*b*) box are continuous through the mesio-occlusal or disto-occlusal parts of the crown.

Features

(*a*) Lock	1.	Extension into fissures.
(Fig. 3.5*a*)	2.	Wide across junction area.
	3.	Shallow; just into dentine.
	4.	Dovetail shape.
	5.	Rounded angles.

(*b*) Box	1.	Walls form a dovetail shape.
(Fig. 3.5*b*)	2.	Axial wall curved across pulp.
	3.	Bevelled axio-pulpal line angle to provide extra thickness of amalgam at weak junction area.
	4.	Laterally extended beyond caries-recurrence area.
	5.	Horizontal cervical finish—no bevel.

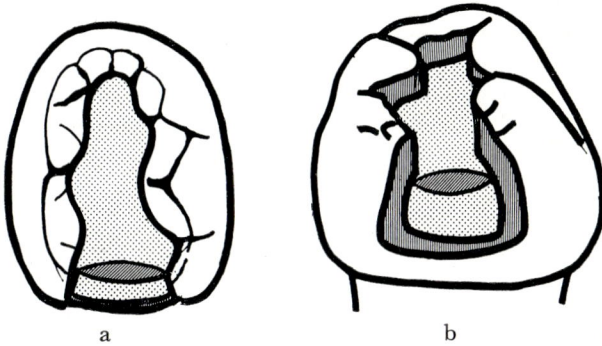

FIG. 3.5.*a* and *b* Diagrams illustrating the preparation of the Class II amalgam cavity. (*a*) The occlusal lock (*b*) The box.

Retention grooves. The pulp of primary molars is most likely to be traumatically exposed at the mesio-lingual and mesio-buccal pulp horns. If this fact is taken into account together with the overall small dimensions of the crown there is a considerable risk in cutting buccal and lingual retention grooves within the box.

The major failure factors in Class II cavities in primary molars are:

1. Lack of width in junctional area between box and key.
2. Lack of bevel on axio-pulpal line angle.
3. Insufficiently large key.

Instrumentation. High-speed airotor burs and diamonds are suitable for forming all main cavity outlines. Primary teeth cut more quickly because of the softer tooth tissue and great care has to be taken when forming the proximal box since damage to the adjacent teeth may easily occur. Bevels such as that of the axio-pulpal line angle, and also the finishing of the cavity outline, should be carried out with the slower speeds.

In Class II cavities the approach is always from the occlusal surface extending the cut into the carious proximal tissue. This method allows a good orientation with regard to cavity depth and there is less risk of accidental pulp exposure than when the primary cut is made in the proximal area.

Matrices. The purpose of a matrix band is to provide a firm contouring surface against which the amalgam may be packed. If it is to perform its function satisfactorily it must fit tightly at the gingival margin, supported by wooden or silver wedges so that a cervical ledge of amalgam is prevented. Once the cavity has been packed, it must be capable of easy release from the tooth, and unless this operation can be completed without disturbance, the setting restoration may be fractured. Choice of matrix band and holder should therefore be governed by the following considerations:

1. Adequate band width so that it can extend below the cervical margin of the box.
2. Correct gauge—0·15 mm so that it can contour easily to the crown shape as the matrix holder is tightened.
3. The matrix holder should have a simple release mechanism so that the band can be left *in situ* for its careful, independent removal once the holder has been taken away. If the holder tightens the band through a system of closed channels both will have to be removed together with a considerable risk to the proximal part of restoration.

Amalgam. The high quality of modern silver amalgams leaves no place for the use of copper amalgam in pedodontics. Claims as to its bacteriocidal properties and its ability to set in the presence of saliva are not good reasons for its use and the emphasis should be placed on improved cavity preparation, improved diet, and saliva control. Five factors are necessary to bring out the excellent qualities of silver amalgam, and they are:

1. Correct cavity preparation.
2. Firmly wedged matrix.
3. Freedom from saliva contamination whilst packing.
4. The amalgam should be tightly packed using automatic packers where possible.
5. Marginal ridges carved down so that they are out of contact with opposing teeth when in occlusion.

Treatment of grossly carious primary molars

Extensive loss of crown substance means that conventional Class II cavity preparation is not possible. Restoration of the tooth in these cases can be achieved only by the use of a preformed crown. The preparation is simple because much of the crown bulk has already been reduced by caries; the remaining surfaces may be quickly shaped. Since the metal crown has to be inserted to an accurate cervical fit, any remaining undercuts due to the anatomical

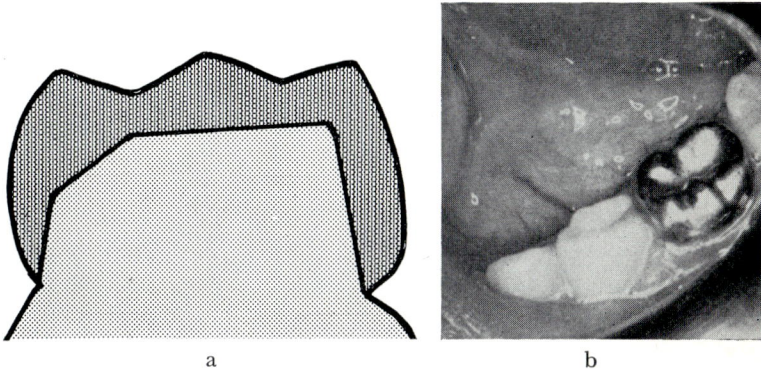

Fig. 3.6a and b. Diagram and photograph of the molar preformed stainless steel crown.
(a) Preparation showing crown tissue scheduled for removal.
(b) Completed crown in the mouth.

shape of the crown mesio-distally, lingually or buccally will require reduction with high-speed burs (Fig. 3.6a, b). The occlusal height of the tooth is then reduced by at least 1mm to accommodate the thickness of the new metal shell without traumatic disturbance against the opposing tooth. Commercially produced steel crowns are available in packs of graded sizes. The size of crown is chosen by measuring with callipers the greatest mesio-distal dimension at the cervical margin of the preparation and relating this to the selection chart in the manufacturer's instructions. The appropriate metal crown is contoured until it fits snugly at the gingival margin, and the rim finally adapted with contouring pliers before polishing the cut edges. The occlusal contact is checked and the crown finally placed in position with zinc phosphate cement.

Inlays. One of the traditional restorations of paedodontics is an inlay described by Willett and designed specifically to restore primary molars with early interproximal caries. The cavity preparation is a proximal slice connected to a T-shaped occlusal slot which provides the retention for the inlay. The time taken to cut the cavity and the amount of tooth tissue removed are similar to that required for the conventional Class II cavity. The advantages of carrying out multiple preparations during the same visit are more theoretical than practical expecially when it is remembered that meisal drift is likely to occur once the contact areas are removed by slicing and that it is difficult to retain temporary dressings in these cavities. There is also need for additional time to record impressions and in the laboratory, for casting and polishing the inlay before it is inserted at the following visit.

Restoration of primary canines

The cavity consists of a labial or palatally cut key which is continuous with the proximal box.

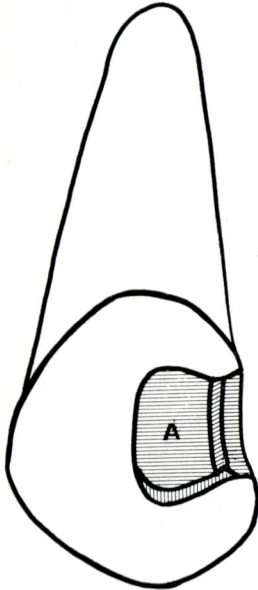

FIG. 3.7. Diagram showing outline of Class III amalgam cavity preparation in a primary canine. The retentive key-way (A) may be cut either on the labial or palatal surface of the crown.

Features (Fig. 3.7)

(*a*) Keyway   1. Shallow.
2. Broad and dovetail shaped.
3. Broad junction area between keyway and box.
4. May be cut on labial or lingual surfaces.

   (*b*) Box   1. Preserve three walls of box if possible.
                 2. Do not extend near to incisal edge as this greatly weakens the tooth at this point and it easily converts, unfavourably to a Class IV cavity.
                 3. Broad junction area between box and keyway.

Matrix and packing. The free matrix band is wedged at the cervical margin and supported either lingually or labially with a piece of warmed compound impression material which is adapted to provide a firm base against adjacent teeth. Silver amalgam is the material of choice for the restoration since its strength and durability are more important than its lack of aesthetic qualities in the primary canine. It is packed into the keyway and box with an automatic condenser, trimmed and finished with polishing strips and sandpaper disks on a subsequent visit.

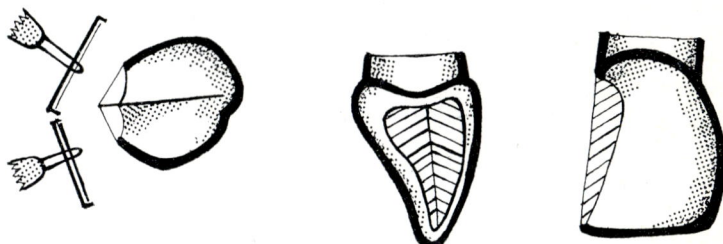

Fig. 3.8. Diagram illustrating the method of discing for proximal caries in primary incisors.
The use of disc guards is essential.

Restoration of primary incisors

Class III cavities can seldom be confined to the proximal surfaces and caries removal leaves the incisal edge weakened so that fracture of the tip frequently occurs. The small crown bulk does not allow room for the addition of a retentive keyway and the following are the methods of treating incisors after caries removal:

(*a*) *Discing* (Fig. 3.8). If the disc cuts are angled into the proximal space the area is made self-cleansing by removing only the minimal amount of crown tissue; thus resulting appearances are poor.

(*b*) *Stainless steel bands* (Fig. 3.9). Either commercial or constructed tailor-made to fit the crown are useful especially when both mesial and distal surfaces are weakened by caries. The bands are cemented in position and left in place as a permanent restoration.

(*c*) *Preformed stainless steel crowns* are produced commercially and these are cemented in position after they have been trimmed cervically in a manner similar to that already described for primary molars.

Treatment of children with rampant caries

There can be few conditions other than rampant caries which show more clearly the inseparable relationship between disease and patient. Success in treatment requires that the operator shall

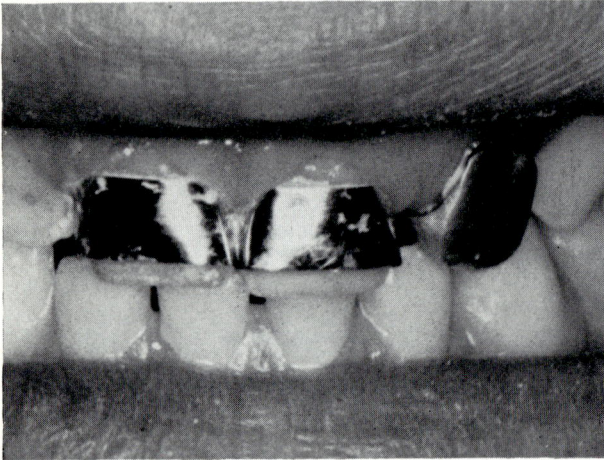

Fig. 3.9. Stainless steel bands cemented on A/A to support crowns weakened by extensive caries.

approach the problem as a total situation. The plan he devises should be based not on theoretical possibilities but on practical details of the child's personality, cooperation and the cumulative dental destruction that has occurred.

In the upper incisor area for example, an acute abscess of a grossly carious incisor may require its extraction, but if adjacent incisors also show gross caries with periapical bone changes, they should be considered for extraction at the same time and their replacements included on the inevitable prosthesis. If any of these teeth required treatment, either singly or in small groups, in an otherwise well cared for mouth, their prognosis would be much improved, since time and cooperation would allow for the appropriate endodontic and restorative measures.

Endodontic treatment of carious teeth

The operator will find himself faced with a limited number of alternative procedures when the pulp has been exposed by the caries or during its excavation. If the pulp is vital it can be (*a*) capped, (*b*) partly removed from the exposure site or (*c*) completely extirpated. The selection of any of these methods depends on the age, dental development, shape of the canal, the initial area of pulp exposure and the method by which the crown will be restored both immediately and eventually. Where the pulp cannot be tested due to extensive crown destruction it should be judged from symptoms

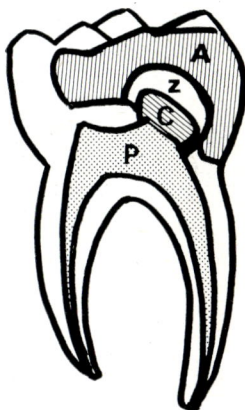

Fig. 3.10. Diagram of pulp capping for an exposed vital pulp in a primary molar
Key: A = Amalgam
    Z = Zinc phosphate cement
    C = Calcium hydroxide paste
    P = Pulp

and the clinical appearance of freshly bleeding tissue at the exposure site and also from periapical radiographs. If there is evidence on the radiograph of periapical disturbance be it periapical bone loss or increase in thickness of associated periodontal ligament then the pulp can no longer be considered normal. The presence of an abnormal pulp makes its partial conservation a doubtful procedure and total extirpation is the method of treatment preferred.

In teeth where the pulp is infected or necrotic as a result of carious exposure, evidence of periapical disturbances is usually found on the radiograph and complete pulp extirpation is essential. Endodontic measures in primary molars are restricted to (*a*) vital pulp capping or (*b*) pulp extirpation when the pulp is necrotic followed by pulp chamber and limited canal filling with zinc oxide-eugenol.

Methods. INITIAL PULP CAPPING. Isolate the tooth and remove all soft caries and dry the exposure surface with sterile cotton pledgets. A small bead of calcium hydroxide paste is placed over the exposure and covered with a layer of zinc phosphate cement and amalgam (Fig. 3.10).

MUMMIFICATION OF THE PULP. This method is useful where the pulp is cariously exposed. The cavity preparation is completed under local anaesthesia and the coronal pulp extirpated by cutting away the roof of the chamber and removing the enclosed tissue with a sharp dentine excavator. Devitalising paste contains the following drugs:

Paraformaldehyde 1·00 g (active devitalising drug)
Lignocaine 0·08 g (anaesthetic)
Carmine 0·50 mg (for colour contrast)
Propylene glycol 0·75 ml. ⎫ to improve working
Carbowax 1·50 g ⎬ consistency

A layer of the paste is placed in the pulp chamber, over the mouths of the canals and sealed in with a layer of phosphate cement. However, it may need to be repeated on a second visit if devitalisation is incomplete.

Ultimately the remaining pulp tissue in the canals becomes mummified, but evidence of this usually has to depend on the absence of symptoms and satisfactory radiographic appearance of the periapical tissues.

Occasionally the paste may be used without removing the coronal pulp, but applied directly to a traumatic pulp exposure. It is less effective in this situation, since the paraformaldehyde frequently causes pain and repeated applications are necessary to achieve pulp mummification.

On rare occasions its use has been suggested for permanent teeth when the pulp vitality is doubtful and where routine endodontic therapy cannot be carried out because of abnormal root formation.

The paste has also been used to devitalise and mummify exposed pulps in haemophiliacs because it does not require a local anaesthetic and no bleeding occurs from the pulp.

The authors do not recommend its use on these occasions as a form of permanent treatment, since in all but deciduous teeth, any technique which does not involve a biochemical cleansing of necrotic tissue in the root canals is not likely to be safe or successful.

WHERE THE PULP IS NECROTIC. The tooth is isolated, the pulp chamber opened up and its necrotic contents removed. Using sterile endodontic instruments, a fine barbed broach is inserted into the root canals so that as much as possible of the radicular pulp remnants are removed. It has to be remembered that these canals are fine and curved, so that reaming is very difficult.

After disinfecting the canals with monochlorphenol they are filled with a calcium hydroxide and iodoform (equal parts by weight) mixed with sterile water and placed in a syringe kept specifically for the purpose. Alternatively, proprietary brands of calcium hydroxide are available in syringe cartridges supplied with broad blunt-ended needles (proprietary name—Reogan Rapid, manufactured by Vivadent-Schaan, Liechtenstein). When the canals are filled with calcium hydroxide, the excess is cleared from the cavity and the floor sealed with a layer of zinc phosphate cement. The amalgam restoration is inserted as soon as the cavity preparation has been completed (Fig. 3.11).

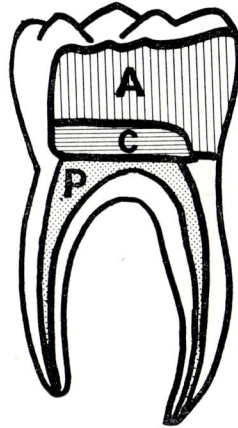

Fig. 3.11. Endondotic treatment of a
primary molar
Key: A = Amalgam
C = Zinc phosphate cement
P = Absorbable paste

Since root canal therapy on primary incisors may result in injury to the underlying developing permanent incisors crowns it should be avoided, and the primary incisors extracted if their pulps are affected.

Endodontics in permanent molars with carious exposures

The first permanent molars are important units in each arch, and become even more so if other teeth, e.g. the $\overline{5/5}$ are missing from the normal series. Under certain circumstances therefore it may be very desirable to preserve such teeth. Furthermore there is a good case for restoring very carious $\underline{6/6}$, as a temporary measure whilst these teeth are providing the main anchorage for an upper removable orthodontic appliance, until $\underline{7/7}$ have erupted. The temporarily retained $\underline{6/6}$ can then be extracted to create space for alignment of other teeth in the arch (see Chapter 7).

Once the pulp has been cariously exposed, the type of endodontic treatment required depends on whether the pulp is vital, and the degree of maturity of the apices.

Vital pulp exposure and immature roots. If, on investigation the pulp is found to be vital, every attempt should be made to preserve its vitality, at least until the apices have matured. The method of choice is the same as that already described for pulp-capping deciduous molars, but teeth treated by this method should be kept under observation and radiographic review every three months for a two-year period.

Sometimes a large pulp exposure site may occur when carious dentine has been removed carelessly. Such cases are not suitable for pulp-capping and their treatment should consist of providing local anaesthesia, isolating the tooth, completing the cavity preparation, cleansing and drying. The whole of the pulp chamber roof is then cut away with burs and the contents removed as far as the root canals. During this stage of treatment it is important to assess the quality of the pulp tissue, whether it is pale and perhaps friable or, on the other hand, whether it bleeds extensively during removal, indicating its hyperaemic condition. Where such changes are apparent, the prognosis for the remaining pulp within the canals is poor and the dentist should consider whether his treatment should include the total removal of pulpal tissue from the tooth. However, if the condition of the pulp seems satisfactory, the treatment can proceed by washing out the cavity with sterile normal saline, drying it, and placing a thick layer of calcium hydroxide paste (Reogan Rapid) over the trimmed pulp amputation stumps at the entrance to the root canals. This is then covered with a layer of quick-setting zinc oxide and eugenol paste followed by zinc phosphate cement and a routine amalgam restoration.

Exposure of non-vital pulp where roots are immature. The treatment of young permanent molars with necrotic pulp tissue, is difficult because of wide, curved root canals with open apices. There is also the problem of obtaining good access where there is restricted opening of the mouth, especially when the child is uncooperative. The treatment is based on rubber dam isolation, and cavity preparation followed by the total removal of the pulp tissue, and a thorough cleansing of the chamber and canal walls with sterile normal saline. The canals are dried and paper points carrying monochlorophenol are inserted as a dressing and sealed into the tooth temporarily with zinc oxide and eugenol filling. If there is a discharge in the canals, then root-filling should be delayed until they are clear and dry. The root-filling may be carried out using a calcium hydroxide/iodoform mixture (proprietary name—Kri paste, manufactured by Pharmachemie, A.G., 8053, Zurich, Switzerland) made into a paste. This is injected from a syringe into the root canals until they are entirely filled. It is often an advantage to include a radio-opaque material in the paste since this indicates whether the canal has been filled in the apical third. Sometimes it is necessary to use a lentulo spiral root-filler in order to carry the paste sufficiently far up the canals. When the calcium hydroxide comes into contact with vital tissue in the developing apices, an intense necrotic reaction takes place at the surface as a result of the high alkalinity (pH 12) of the paste. Eventually a layer of scar tissue forms in the contact area and this then calcifies so that adjacent vital tissue will promote a further maturing of the root apices. The remainder of the crown is filled as previously described.

If symptoms, such as pain, swelling and tenderness to percussion develop, together with radiographic evidence of periapical bone loss then extraction of the tooth is the most suitable treatment. On the other hand, if the treated tooth continues to be symptomless and shows radiographically that there is a well-formed lamina dura around the completed apices it should be kept under routine surveillance until standard root canal therapy can be carried out. It is important to realise that the bacteriological status of such teeth cannot be assured, and where the child develops a disease such as rheumatic fever he is endangered by hidden foci of infection in the body. Under these and similar circumstances the doubtful teeth should be extracted as soon as possible with a suitable antibotic cover (see Chapter 6).

4 Treatment of Soft Tissue Lesions

The soft tissues may be injured by trauma, by infection, or they may reflect changes due to drugs or alteration in their ability to heal, as in blood dyscrasias.

Teething

Teething episodes are often more severe when the child has an upper respiratory infection or a common cold. Under these circumstances the fall in tissue resistance may allow local oral infection to occur and increase the child's general feeling of malaise.

Local treatment. The irritation may cause the child to chew any hard object which he can put into his mouth and this helps to break down the overlying gum tissue and release the crowns. Surgical incision of the overlying gum is advised only in exceptional circumstances, since it introduces the risk of infection into the crypt especially if the tooth is still some way from eruption.

The topical application of a surface anaesthetic such as lignocaine ointment will greatly relieve pain before feeding and sleeping, but should be applied sparingly to the teething area so as not to cause distress by anaesthetising the tongue. Where local infection occurs, it should be treated topically:

> *3 per cent Aureomycin* in 10 per cent glycerine applied as a paint to affected areas of the mouth before meals over a period of five days.

General treatment. Loss of sleep is an additional burden to both child and parents. In the very young, aspirin may be given as a suspension or mixed with food or milk:

> *Junior Aspirin:* 1 tablet 80 mg (0-6 months)
> 2 tablets 160 mg (7 months-3 years).

If the pain becomes very severe the following should be prescribed:

> *Paracetamol Elixir Paediatric:*
>
> 5 ml (up to age of 1 year)
> 10 ml (1-5 years.).

Since pyrexia and excessive salivation lead to fluid loss the liquid intake should be increased.

If moniliasis (Thrush) is present then Nystatin should be given (for dosage see under section on *Thrush*).

Pericoronitis

Inflammation of the gum surrounding erupting teeth especially $\frac{6|6}{6|6}$ is common and is often associated with traumatic injury to overlying soft tissues as opposing teeth move towards occlusion. Injury, local infection and stagnation in the molar region may produce a swollen operculum.

Unlike the condition in lower 3rd molars, the situation is temporary and will disappear when the $\frac{6|6}{6|6}$ erupt, so that frequent hot salt mouthwashes are usually the only treatment that is required. Where severe pain is experienced however the mouthwash should be followed by the use of local anaesthetic ointment applied at mealtimes and, concurrently, soluble aspirin may be administered. Tooth-brushing in the affected area will not be possible until the pain has subsided and for the same reason the child should change to a soft diet.

Acute ulcero-membranous stomatitis (Vincent's infection)

Local treatment. Immediate treatment begins with a gentle mouth cleansing using hydrogen peroxide, 10/vol. on cotton rolls. Even though the gums are extremely painful, frothing produced by the solution rapidly clears debris from the gingivae so that an improvement is soon felt. The patient is asked to continue with the same strength hydrogen peroxide in frequent mouthwashes at home and to return the following day for preliminary scaling of supra-gingival calculus. The condition rapidly improves with the use of the oxidising mouthwash; in two to three days the pain has gone completely. However, there is a tendency for relapse unless gingival irritation and stagnation areas are removed.

General treatment. If regional lymph nodes become swollen and there is general malaise, systemic penicillin should be given by mouth:

Phenoxymethylpenicillin (Penicillin V):
　　　　　62·5 mg (up to 1 year)
　　　　　125 mg (1-14 years)
　　　　　250 mg (14 years onwards)
　　　　　Four times daily for 5 days.

Aspirin or paracetamol are given to control the pain in the early stages and an increase in fluid intake is required to replace loss by excessive salivation. Home care includes burning the patient's old toothbrush and avoiding contact with other peoples washing and feeding utensils. A soft diet should be provided with increased vitamin supplements, e.g. Adexalin (contains vitamins A and D), and Haliborange (vitamin C). When symptoms have subsided, a new soft toothbrush and a supervised cleansing technique will be required.

Acute bacterial infection

A streptococcal stomatitis or gingivitis in children occurs only rarely although the infection may be localised where tissue is damaged or where resistance is poor.

Local treatment. Hot salt mouthwashes combined with local cleansing of stagnation areas and scaling are usually sufficient to improve the situation.

General treatment. Systemic antibiotics may be necessary if regional lymph nodes become enlarged and malaise becomes serious:

> *Phenoxymethylpenicillin* (Pencillin V)
> *Dose:* see previous section.

Moniliasis (Thrush)

It is essentially a disease of infancy but debilitated or diabetic adult patients may be affected. Thrush sometimes occurs in patients who are on systemic antibiotic therapy (see section on drugs in Chapter 2). In the very young the infection may arise from contaminated nipples or from feeding-bottle teats which have been used without proper cleansing.

Nystatin can be used topically or systemically:

> *Nystatin mixture B.P.C.* (Nystatin 100,000 units in 1 ml):
> 1 ml every 6 hours for 5 days (up to 5 years).
> *In older children* (6-12 years.) Nystatin tablets B.P.C.:
> 1,000,000 units in divided doses daily;
> 2-3 tablets daily for 5 days.

Treatment should include improvement in cleanliness of feeding conditions and eliminating other possible sources of infection.

Acute herpetic gingivostomatitis

Local treatment. 3 per cent Aureomycin in 10 per cent glycerine is used as a paint applied to affected areas for 5 days, three times daily before meals.

Occasionally, local areas of moniliasis may develop and should be treated as already described. Removal of debris and supragingival calculus should be carried out and a local anaesthetic ointment applied to the sore ulcerated areas especially before meals.

General treatment. Pain is controlled by aspirin or paracetamol and the fluid intake is increased. If there is a severe infection with involvement of regional lymph nodes and marked malaise, the systemic antibiotics by mouth should be prescribed to reduce secondary infection.

Traumatic ulcers

These may arise as a result of traumatic injury, or where the lips are irritated against an orthodontic appliance.

Local treatment. They are usually resolved by applying Adcortyl in Orabase (Triamcinolone dental paste, Squibb) and removing the source of irritation.

Puberty gingivitis and poor lip seal

Hormonal changes occurring during puberty may result in a marginal gingivitis which may become severe if oral hygiene is neglected. Local measures such as scaling and polishing followed by an improvement in toothbrushing is usually sufficient. However, the gingival changes associated with poor lip seal are less easily corrected. If the lips are potentially competent, that is prevented from normal tooth coverage only because of malocclusion, then orthodontic treatment will improve the situation. However, the lip position in Class II division 1 cases will nearly always show some improvement after orthodontic treatment so that the child who needs to posture in order to obtain a lip seal will do so more easily when the position of the teeth is more favourable.

Local treatment of the gingival tissue is similar to that for puberty gingivitis except that with the additional drying factor due to lip shortness treatment needs to be more continuous with greater attention to oral hygiene.

Acute Dental Abscess

Presentation

When confined within bone the acute abscess causes severe pain, usually of a throbbing and continuous character. There is tenderness of the related non-vital tooth which is often carious and slightly loose. Occasionally the offending tooth may be fractured or recently filled. There may be some hyperaemia of the immediately related soft tissues at this stage and the patient, particularly the younger child, is often febrile, fractious and off-colour.

It may be a matter of hours or days before the overlying cortical bone is perforated, after which one can expect a facial or other soft-tissue swelling. These usually appear directly related to the tooth involved, but occasionally, as in the case of the infected upper lateral incisor, the abscess may track backwards towards the soft palate before it presents as a painful swelling. When there is a release of intra-bony pressure the pain usually eases at this stage. The rate of increase in facial swelling in the smaller child may be dramatic, particularly in the soft tissues over the maxilla, where a very large swelling can arise in a matter of a few hours.

Submandibular abscesses more commonly arise from breakdown of inflamed lymph nodes rather than by direct spread from the periapical region of related teeth. Frequently there is no adequate dental cause for an abscess in this area in children, and invasion is sometimes never satisfactorily determined.

Management

The history is of great importance. In particular, an assessment of the likelihood of the presence of a significant amount of pus will be more accurate if the clinician knows the duration of the swelling and of any current antibiotic therapy. On this information he can base his decision as to whether incision and drainage will be required. Other points of particular specific importance in this context include trismus, pyrexia, dysphagia, dyspnoea and general malaise.

The clinical examination when facial swelling is present involves extraoral and intraoral components and is proceeded with in the standard fashion (inspection, palpation and percussion).

The distribution, colour and consistency of the soft-tissue swelling is noted together with the presence or absence of tenderness. Intra-orally, the extent of any trismus that might be present is noted. In particular, of course, the presence of carious, loose or tender teeth in relation to the soft-tissue swelling or to its field of lymphatic drainage are noted. Swelling, reddening and tenderness of the soft tissues, particularly over the outer aspect of the alveolar ridge in relation to the causative tooth, may be present. Occasionally pus may ooze from a sinus through the mucosa over the outer alveolar plate or through the gingival sulcus and, where possible, a swab from the area should be sent for bacteriological examination and antibiotic sensitivities.

Swelling of the floor of the mouth or of the lateral wall of the pharynx together with the presence of marked trismus or dysphagia or dyspnoea have serious implications as regards the patency of the airway and should usually be considered for immediate referral to hospital. If the patient is very toxic, a period of twelve or twenty-four hours should be devoted to controlling the toxaemia by antibiotic therapy and to rehydration before surgical treatment is undertaken. Consultation with a paediatrician on general supportive measures at this stage is desirable. If toxaemia is not marked, arrangements may be made for any necessary surgical treatment at once. Usually, where an abscess arises in relation to a deciduous tooth, extraction is indicated. For permanent teeth, of course, extraction or, alternatively, drainage via the pulp canal, with subsequent root canal therapy, may be indicated.

In either case, where a significant amount of pus is present in the soft tissues, incision and drainage are required. Depending on the area involved this may be carried out by an extraoral or an intraoral approach. Extraoral drainage is most often necessary for submandibular abscessess and is usually carried out in hospital. An attempt is made to site the skin incision so that when the swelling has resolved, the scar will lie parallel to and about 1-2 cm below the lower border of the mandible. After the skin incision has been made a pair of sinus or artery forceps are introduced between the fibres of the platysma muscle into the collection of pus. The forceps are then opened and withdrawn, thereby creating a pathway for the release of the pus (Hilton's method) (Fig. 4.1 a, b). A suitable drain is introduced into the abscess cavity and retained for twenty-four to forty-eight hours until drainage has ceased.

Intraoral drainage, usually employed for facial rather than for, submandibular or submental abscesses, is usually carried out by incision in the line of the reflection of the buccal or labial sulcus. The gravitational element is, of course, unfavourable in the lower jaw, but the technique avoids the necessity for a facial skin incision and is usually successful.

Where possible, a specimen of pus is sent for bacteriological

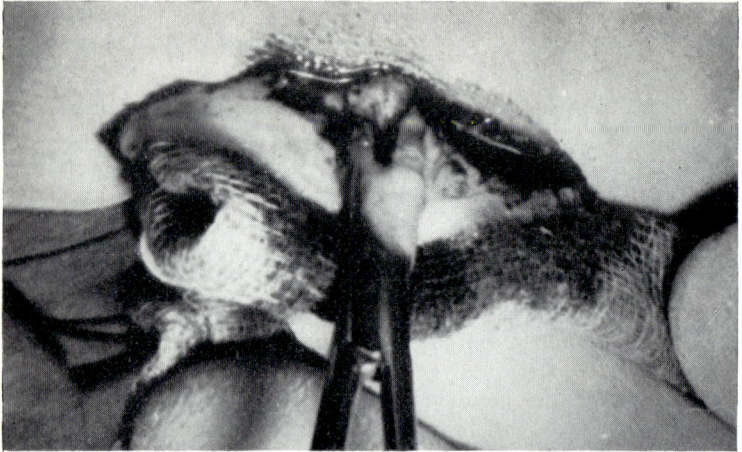

a

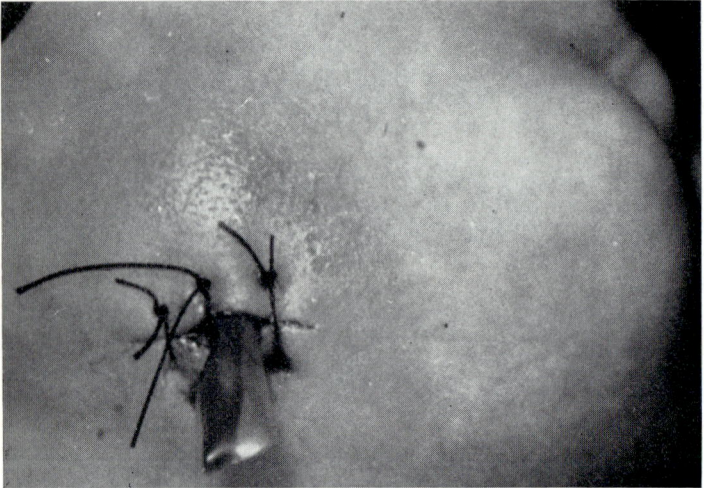

b

Fig. 4.1.*a* and *b* (*a*) Extraoral incision to establish drainage
(*b*) External drain in position.

investigation and is used to determine the sensitivity of organisms
to the concurrent use of antibiotics. During the acute phase, and
until the sensitivities were available, the antibiotic initially used
would be benzylpenicillin (by injection 300 mg four times a day; and
then phenoxymethylpenicillin 125-250 mg four times a day by
mouth for five days to maintain the blood level of antibiotics).

The differential diagnosis must be made from swellings of non-dental origin including mumps, and especially when involving the submandibular salivary glands, sialadenitis secondary to sialectasis (more commonly involving the parotid gland in childhood), and submandibular lymphadenopathy (usually detected by bimanual palpation with the forefinger of the left hand placed in the floor of the mouth). Ranula involving the floor of the mouth or the ventral surface of the tongue, is usually easily distinguished from inflammatory involvement of these areas.

Complications

Infection in the upper anterior teeth may become extensive and spreading in character so that an orbital cellulitis rapidly develops. In such circumstances there is a risk of the infection passing through the median vein of the orbit, producing a fatal cavernous sinus thrombosis. Where there are indications that the cellulitis is moving towards this stage then immediate hospital supervision and surgical relief are necessary, usually by extraction of the offending tooth, sometimes accompanied by an incision in the labial sulcus as already mentioned. Benzylpenicillin is given by injection immediately (300 mg) and repeated every six hours until the initial acute stage is passed and the patient is then maintained on Phenoxymethyl-penicillin (penicillin V) 250 mg by mouth every six hours for five to seven days.

Treatment of abscessed primary teeth

An acute abscess of the primary dentition nearly always means that the extraction of the tooth is essential. Where the acute stage has subsided into a chronic phase there is an attempt on the part of the tissues to localise the inflammatory area which periodically discharges through a sinus. It is at this stage that the pulp chamber of the abscessed tooth may be opened up, once it has been isolated, and its necrotic contents together with those from the canals removed as far as possible. Because of the fineness of the canals and the root curvature in the molars, only limited use of broaches and fine reamers is possible. Paper points soaked in monochlorphenol or beechwood cresote are inserted into the chamber and canals to provide an antiseptic coating to the walls. They are then filled with a calcium hydroxide mixture from a syringe and capped with cement and amalgam (see Chapter 3). In many cases the persistence of a chronic apical lesion is due to gradual release of necrotic and

E

infected pulp products from the canal into the periapical tissues. Once the canal has been cleared, the apical tissues gradually return to normal and the sinus disappears leaving a tooth which is functional and only rarely subject to ankylosis. Such treatment is indicated only in those mouths where the chronic dental abscess is an isolated occurrence and where there are no health hazards. If many such teeth are present they should be extracted.

Where endodontic treatment has been carried out, a periodic radiographic check is necessary to ensure that the periapical condition is satisfactory. Whilst this limited form of root canal therapy is successful on primary molars it is not recommended for primary incisors because of the risk to the underlying developing permanent crowns, defects of which will eventually effect the appearance at the front of the mouth.

Abscesses of permanent teeth

The factors which govern the treatment are:

The acuteness of the condition
The medical complications that might arise as a result of sepsis.
The tooth involved, its maturity and the possibility of treating the canal satisfactorily.
Satisfactory periodontal support.

In some cases, because of severe arch crowding or local imbrication it may benefit the patient to have the tooth extracted. When incisors are involved, the result of their loss is considered in Chapter 7. It is usually unnecessary to extract these teeth as they are accessible for root canal therapy and apical root resection, should the latter become necessary. Molar and premolar teeth are not always successfully treated because of curved roots, inaccessible canals and problems with isolation during treatment. They may therefore require extraction if an acute abscess occurs.

Establishing drainage. An acute abscess of a permanent incisor requires immediate drainage if the tooth is to be retained. Unfortunately the situation is not easily resolved because the patient is suffering severe throbbing pain and the tooth is very tender to the touch. The accumulation of inflammatory fluids may be so great in the periodontal ligament that the tooth is displaced from its normal incisal position and interferes with the occlusion. Facial swelling, pyrexia, general malaise and enlarged regional lymph nodes may also add to the discomfort. Infiltrations of local anaesthetic solution in the abscess area are contraindicated because of the risk of spreading the infection. The dental surgeon must decide, therefore, whether it is necessary for the patient to receive a general anaesthetic in order to establish drainage although in the majority of cases this is not necessary and with patience, a highspeed round diamond bur can quickly cut through to the pulp chamber. Vibration and discomfort are greatly reduced if the tooth is gently steadied with a composition splint whilst the airotor is cutting the crown. Pus may gush forth from the canal once it is opened, or alternatively there may be no immediate relief of pressure so that the canal contents must be cleared with a barbed broach before drainage can be established. Rubber dam is not used in the initial painful stage, but it is advisable once the drainage has been successful.

The patient is immediately relieved from severe pain once drainage has become established and is asked to use hot salt mouthwashes frequently for the following twenty-four hours during which time the canal is left open for the escape of fluids. If no drainage can be established by the root canal it is possible to attempt direct surgical drainage under general anaesthesia by incision over the apical abscess. However, this will only be successful if the swelling is localised and if this method fails, extraction of the incisor is the only realistic solution. Analgesics, e.g. aspirin or paracetamol will be required (see under *Teething*).

Treatment of infected extraction sockets

The variety of factors which may be responsible for the infection of a socket include (*a*) retained roots; (*b*) the vasoconstriction effect of the adrenalin in the local anaesthetic solution; (*c*) incorrect extraction technique in which considerable bruising occurs in the bony sockets walls and surrounding soft tissues, so that their ability to form a satisfactory blood clot is impaired. Occasionally an extraction may tear the surrounding mucosa and prolonged bleeding in the area causes a large unstable clot. Poor healing may be encountered as part of a generalised debility or if the child carries a systemic infection, but, however, it should be remembered that failure of the tissues to respond adequately to injury may be the first indication that the child is suffering from a form of blood dyscrasia.

Local treatment. Examination, including radiographs, of the socket should be carried out to determine the extent to which local factors such as retained roots or mucosal tears are responsible for the painful socket. Any remaining clot should be carefully removed and if necessary rough bone margins are reduced with bone rongeurs and the mucosa sutured back over the socket margins under local anaesthesia.

A dirty, fragmenting blood clot accompanied by severe pain, marked halitosis, trismus and sometimes swelling all indicate an infection of the socket. It is unusual in children to find the socket completely devoid of clot ('dry socket'). The socket should be gently syringed with about 40 ml of warm Dakin's solution until all the clot fragments are washed clear. A zinc oxide/eugenol pack is inserted gently and aspirin is recommended to control the pain. Systemic penicillin (phenoxymethylpenicillin: for dosage see under *Treatment of Vincent's infection*) may be given by mouth if the infection is extending or if malaise becomes marked. Frequent hot saline mouthwashes will assist the healing locally, but the socket will usually require irrigation with Dakin's solution for two to three days accompanied by replacement of zinc oxide/eugenol packs. If there is any suspicion that the healing is unduly delayed the child should be referred for haematological investigation.

Eruption cysts

The condition may vary from a well-established cyst which may be difficult to differentiate from an early dentigerous cyst, to a blue haematoma formed in the overlying mucosa which is the result of trauma before eruption occurs. It is probable that the majority belong to the latter group.

Treatment. Since the eruption cyst tends to resolve as it is decompressed traumatically between the erupting and opposing tooth, there is little treatment required. Attempts at surgical interference should be resisted, since the tooth may not have reached its final pre-eruption position, and premature surgery may allow infection to enter the tooth crypt.

For the treatment of dentigerous cysts the reader is referred to a standard textbook on oral surgery, but the salient factor which should be noticed on the radiograph is whether the relevant tooth is displaced from its eruption site by the expanding cyst.

Mucous Cysts

Mucous cysts sometimes occur in the lips due to a blocking of the orifice of a mucous gland. The condition is characterised by a painless swelling which gradually increases in size.

Treatment consists of enucleation of the cyst or its decompression by passing a suture through the swelling. This allows epithelialisation to occur round the suture and provides permanent drainage.

5 Oral Trauma and Endodontics

Injury to a child's mouth from a blow or a fall is as dramatic as its results are far reaching. In the space of a moment the harmony of the mouth can be destroyed and the child committed to long periods of treatment to recapture the natural appearance. The damage may range from a simple crown fracture to multiple injuries sustained in an automobile accident where dental trauma is of relatively minor concern as cranial and chest wounds compete for emergency treatment.

Even when the child arrives at the surgery some hours after the dental injury has occurred the state of distress is often in evidence. Those severely affected by the episode may show signs of shock such as pale, sweating features, restless hands and apprehension. Added to this is the understandable concern of the parent or teacher, which increases the burden the child has to bear.

The experienced dental surgeon will realise that litigation may arise where the patient has suffered injury as a result of either civil negligence or even juvenile assault, and he will be well advised to ensure adequacy of notes and radiographs as they may be an important factor in later legal proceedings such as the compilation of reports for solicitors.

Predisposing factors

Since oral trauma is so common during childhood it is likely to occur when the infant increases in mobility. As soon as he begins to strive for a more independent existence he embarks on a journey of exploration of surrounding objects such as furniture, doors and chairs. The objectives of his expedition include testing taste, hardness, mobility and spatial relationships of all the obstacles he meets and in so doing he may move into potentially dangerous and unexpected situations where, for example, an opening door may accidently strike him in the face. It is much more common, however, to find that mouth injuries in the very young are due to falls on to steps or against hard chair backs and cot rails. Apart from taking the usual commonsense precautions that most mothers practise, there seems little chance of anticipating many of these accidents.

Sports such as soccer, hockey, boxing and swimming also cause dental trauma in the older child, but the out-of-context, unexpected accident is more commonly responsible for this type of injury. As one would expect, certain seasonal activities increase the risk of injury and these include sleighing, ice-skating, sliding on ice and snow-balling. Poor winter road conditions such as fog and ice make driving and braking hazardous, so that if seat belts are not used dento-facial injuries may occur against unpadded interior fitments.

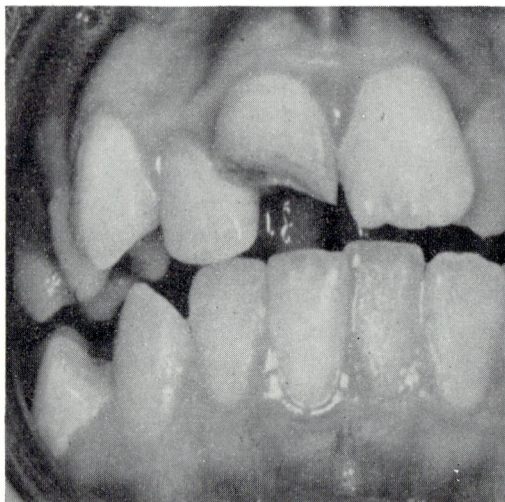

FIG. 5.1. Traumatic injury to a proclined incisor in a mouth which is crowded but basically has a Class I incisal relationship.

Certain intrinsic factors may make the child more liable to dental injury. It is commonly found in the child with a Class II division 1 malocclusion, the proclined upper teeth are more susceptible to injury than those with normal incisor relationships. Factors responsible for this are the greatly increased overjet with little contact between upper and lower incisors and also the characteristically incompetent lips which leave the front teeth exposed to the blow. In a similar way individual incisors which are proclined due to severe local arch crowding may receive the full force of the blow. (Fig. 5.1).

With any defect in the quality of the teeth such as a result of hypo-plasia or dental caries, or where there has been a root filling, post or jacket crown, the tooth is weakened so that fracture may occur following relatively minor trauma.

Facial injuries are particularly common in epileptic children due to falls against hard objects or on to the floor during loss of consciousness. Their special problems with regard to endodontics, jacket crowns and dentures are discussed in Chapter 6.

Factors affecting type of injury

The blow to the mouth can vary in several ways so that a broad classification may help to relate it to the type of injury that it is

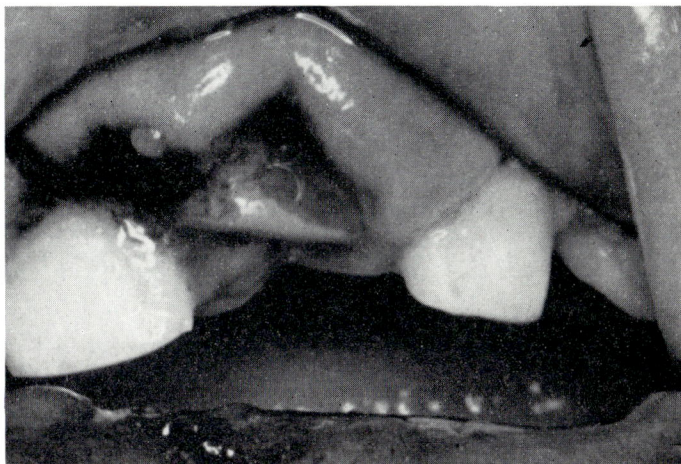

Fig. 5.2. Palatal displacement of A/ by trauma: /A has been intruded into the maxillary alveolus.

likely to produce. The object causing the injury may be considered in the following manner:

1. *Hardness.* A hard, firm substance, such as stone tends to shatter the crown tissue on contact. The fracture line may be restricted to the crown or continue obliquely into the root. If confined to the crown it is often possible to see associated enamel crazing where cracked enamel is still supported by firm dentine (see Chapter 2).

If the injury results from a blow against a relatively soft surface such as a boot or a wooden object, there is a greater tendency to tooth displacement although crown and root fracture may also occur.

2. *Speed.* If the trauma is delivered slowly as when a child's face is pushed against a pavement or fence, the teeth are displaced rather than fractured. On the other hand the stone travelling at high

speed contacts the crown with a sharp hard blow—fracturing it but at the same time causing less direct injury to the root and periapical tissues.

3. *Direction.* Teeth may be pushed upwards (in the case of upper incisors), forwards or backwards (Fig. 5.2) depending on the direction of the blow relative to the position of the head. Displacement of primary incisors is much more common than crown or root fracture. This result is to be expected especially where root resorption has reduced the area of attachment.

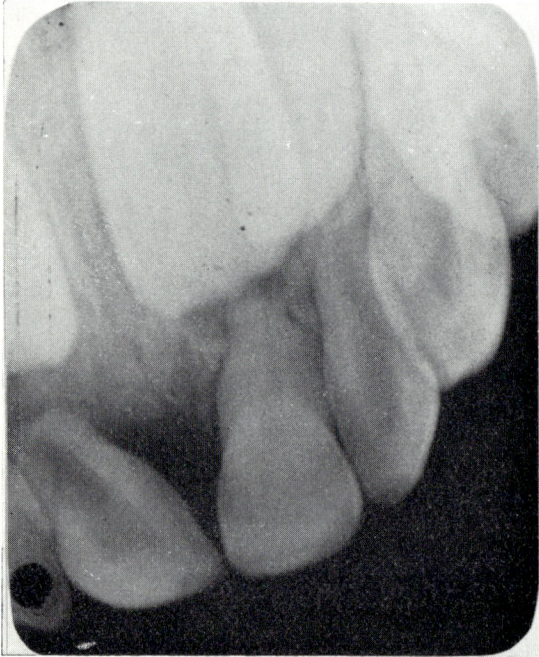

Fig. 5.3. Radiograph showing resorption of A/A roots

Traumatic Injuries to the Primary Dentition

Fractures of the crowns of primary incisors are less commonly found than in the permanent dentition, but displacement more frequently occurs as a result of injury. There are several reasons why this should be so, the first being that the very young child's environment is largely domestic and to some extent protected. His accidents are falls which occur largely from errors in his experimental assessment of his environment; he may misjudge balance, heights and hardness. Secondly, the roots of the primary incisors lie between the developing permanent crowns palatally and a thin plate of bone labially so that resistance to displacement is not so great at this stage especially if resorption of the deciduous roots has already begun (Fig. 5.3).

Types of tooth displacement

Theoretically, although the primary incisors can be displaced in any direction, the commonest forms are intrusion and retroclination.

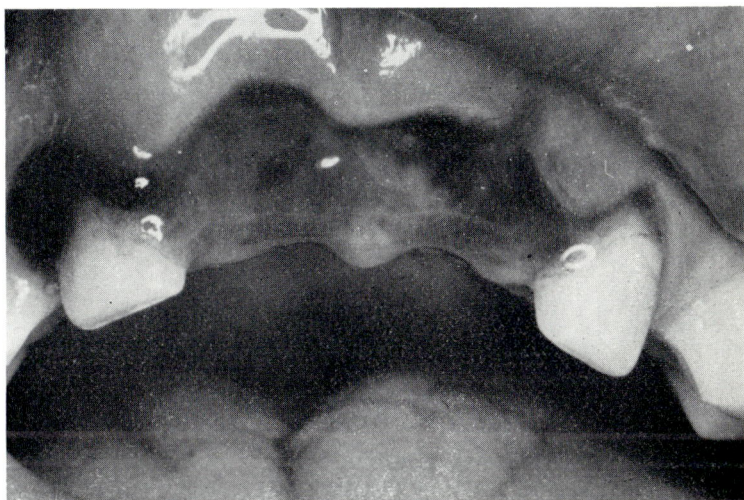

Fig. 5.4. Complete intrusion of A/A following traumatic injury

Intrusion of the upper primary incisors is the result of a fall in which the force of the blow is directed up in the long axis of the tooth. It is not uncommon to find on examination that the tooth has apparently disappeared from the arch. All that may remain is an entry wound covered with blood clot and a bulge in the labial sulcus (Fig. 5.4). The fact that the tooth can be displaced to such an extent is an indication of the flexible arrangement of the tissue surrounding its roots, a feature often disadvantageous to the developing permanent incisor (see *Dilaceration* below).

Confusion may sometimes arise where the primary incisor is thought to have been completely lost, but the tell-tale swelling in the upper labial sulcus together with a periapical radiograph will confirm the presence of the tooth in its displaced position.

Retroclination. The deciduous incisor may be pushed backwards to a position where it interferes with the normal occlusion of the teeth (Fig. 5.5). It is commonly found that as the palatal movement occurs at the time of injury the tooth is carried further out of its socket, exposing part of the root labially. If the root is still full length, a bulge in the labial sulcus will denote the position of the apex tipped outwards against the overlying alveolar structures.

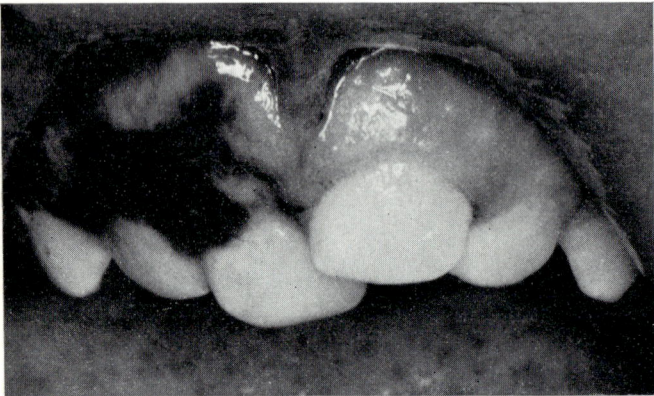

FIG. 5.5. Palatally displaced BA/ preventing centric occlusion.

Root fracture may occur during injury to the primary incisors, but it is not common. It is more likely to take place in the younger age-groups before root absorption had begun.

Sequelae of injury

Pulp necrosis and crown discoloration may occur following relatively minor traumatic episodes without marked tooth displacement. This is found to occur more usually in the younger age-groups and may be followed by a chronic dental abscess and sinus.

However, discoloration of the crown need not always mean the inevitable loss of the tooth, since there is often a spontaneous improvement in colour and return of vitality in the first few weeks following injury. There seems to be little doubt in these cases that the staining within the crown is from the breakdown products of pulp haemorrhage, which appear to be largely resorbed if the pulp tissue survives.

In other circumstances radiographic examination of primary incisors with slight loss in normal translucency may reveal that complete pulp calcification has occurred.

Very often intruded deciduous incisors return down their injury pathway to their original position. However, their apical vascular supply has been severed and they can no longer be regarded as normal teeth even where discoloration has not occurred.

Sequelae in permanent dentition

One of the unfortunate consequences of injury to the primary incisors is the damge that may be transmitted to the related developing permanent teeth. The type of defect found (See Fig. 2.23) in the permanent tooth is usually as a result of either direct trauma to the partly developed permanent crown or to the close proximity of a chronic abscess of a deciduous incisor.

Often a more serious deformity occurs when the crown and perhaps part of the root of a permanent incisor has calcified, but the remainder of the root is in a flexible organic state. Within its bony environment a blow transmitted to the rigid structure will displace it but the incompletely calcified root portion tends to remain in its original position. As eruption eventually occurs, concurrently with the completion of the root the developing angulation in the root (see Fig. 2.10) leads to an abnormal eruption path or even prevents eruption. Unfortunately, root resection is not a possible solution in many of these cases because such a considerable proportion of root is involved.

Trauma to the primary incisors may cause delayed exfoliation because of partial ankylosis with the result that the erupting permanent incisor is deflected palatally. If this occurs in an arch with potential crowding, space reserved for the deflected tooth may be partly taken up by reciprocal drift of adjacent units. However, delayed exfoliation or premature loss of the primary incisors is seldom entirely responsible for malocclusion in the upper labial segments.

Treatment

When the primary incisors are severely injured as when the pulp is exposed or if the roots are fractured, they should be extracted. If one bears in mind the relative proximity of the roots of the primary teeth to the developing crowns of the permanent teeth there is a considerable risk to these structures if root canal therapy of A/A, is undertaken or doubtful periapical conditions allowed to persist.

If A/A are displaced palatally an attempt to reposition them is

likely to disturb the developing 1/1 crowns. Under these circumstances they should be extracted, but often the primary incisors may
be mobile with only minimal displacement. Providing no attempt is
made to reposition them in the arch, they should be splinted (see
later) and their periapical condition periodically reviewed. Upper
primary incisors that have been intruded usually tend to return
gradually to the occlusal plane. However, immediately following
trauma the tooth is lying high up in the flexible environment of the
developing permanent crown and the alveolar tissues, both of which
have been displaced and are under tension as a result of the intrusion.
It is not surprising to find that the pressure exerted against the
inclined surfaces of the deciduous crown produces an effect like an
orange pip between the finger and thumb.

The principles of treating these teeth lie in an appreciation of the
following facts:

(*a*) They carry bacteria into the immediate environment of the
developing permanent crown.

(*b*) Their slow return means that there will be a persistent pathway for infection into the tissues until the incisor has
achieved its previous occlusal level.

(*c*) The periapical vessels of the traumatised primary tooth
cannot survive more than slight displacement and the
vitality of the tooth must, therefore, be lost. Since re-
vitalisation of such pulp tissue cannot be considered a
possibility under these circumstances, whatever the ultimate
position of the tooth, its necrotic pulp is a major factor against
retaining it in the mouth even if infection does not subsequently occur.

Calcification of the pulp sometimes occurs as a result of a degenerative mechanism initiated by the injury. It is found more
commonly in teeth that have suffered little or no displacement and
suggests that such degenerative damage can only take place if there
is still a limited vascular circulation within the pulp. Judging from
the radiographic appearance, there appears to be little periapical
disturbance once the pulp calcification has taken place and the
tooth should, in these circumstances, be allowed to remain but kept
under periodoc observation every six months.

Occasionally the child is brought to the surgery some weeks
following the injury, for example when the tooth discolours, and it is
difficult to make an accurate assessment of the initial degree of
displacement or other injury that has occurred. In these circumstances great reliance should be placed upon radiographic evidence

of an intact periapical lamina dura of the primary incisor, but super-imposition against the underlying permanent crown may make an accurate interpretation difficult.

Traumatic Injuries to Permanent Dentition

Fracture of the crown without direct pulp involvement may consist of enamel crazing where the intact dentine maintains the integrity of the outer cracked enamel shell (see Fig. 2.6). More serious injury may occur, such as a deep fracture passing close to the pulp horns and breaking off as much as one-third of the crown (Fig. 5.6).

Such injuries may show the following features. There is usually pulp disturbance which often appears to be unrelated to the degree

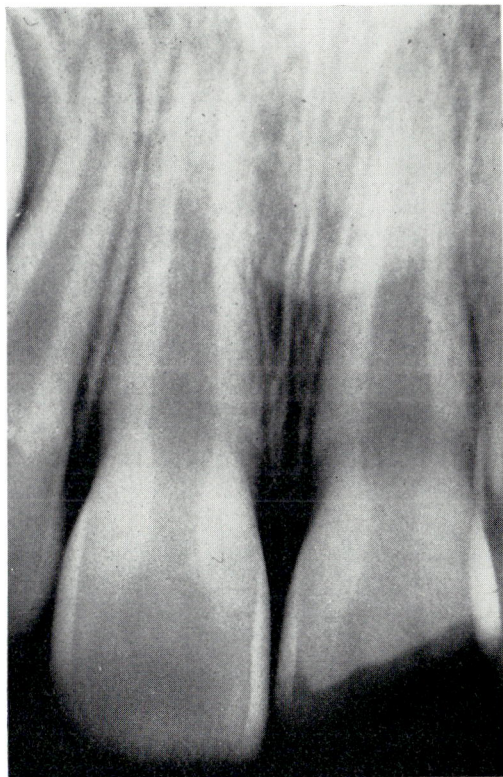

Fig. 5.6. Radiograph showing extensive crown fracture passing close to the pulp horns of a permanent central incisor.

of crown injury. In some cases the teeth after suffering minimal trauma (scarcely recollected by the patient) become non-vital as pulp necrosis occurs. On other occasions degenerative changes similar to those in the primary incisors result in pulp calcification. If the great variation in these responses is taken into account, it seems unwise to make positive predictions based on the apparent

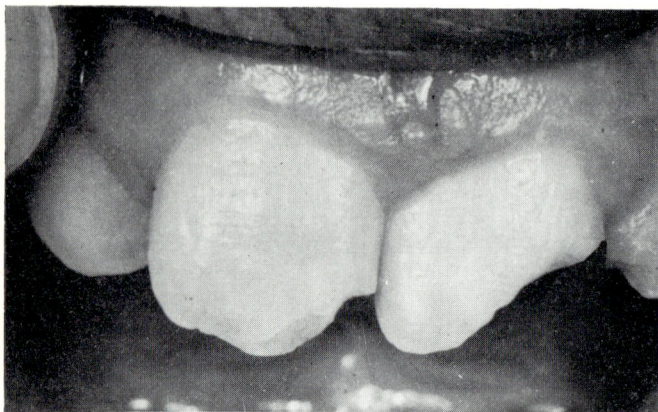

Fig. 5.7. The extent and position of the fracture plane /1 make it difficult for this tooth to retain a temporary protective crown.

degree of tooth injury. It does seem clear, however, that some form of pulp reaction nearly always occurs and may be a purely beneficial stimulation of odontoblasts producing secondary dentine to re-establish the pulp's former isolation from the external environment. The periapical tissues are likely to be involved by tooth movement at the time of injury even though this may mean only a momentary displacement. Where the root of the permanent incisor is immature the large vascular supply into the funnel-shaped apex is unlikely to suffer so much as the restricted blood supply in a completely formed root. Under these circumstances degenerative pulp calcification is more likely to occur where the apical vascular supply has been reduced to its mature level, rather than in the young immature incisor with its wide apex having maximum circulation.

The immediate object of treatment is to protect dentine which is sensitive to chemical and thermal changes. The fractured surface should be covered with a cap which can stand up to wear and tear for ten weeks without need for recementing or remaking. Two of the main causes for losing the protective cap are its tendency to deform and attempting to retain it on a difficult crown fracture (Fig. 5.7).

In the early stages where protection is the main consideration, the appearance is of secondary importance. Nevertheless, certain forms of protective cap such as those made from copper crown rings rapidly become foul and blackened due to reaction with sulphides in the oral cavity and should be avoided if any other form of covering can be provided. It is essential to remember that where there is a degree of crowding in the incisor area, there will be competition for any space that becomes available following loss of crown tissue. In this respect the crown protection should be constructed to such a length that it will prevent the further eruption or proclination of lower incisors, otherwise the subsequent restoration of the fractured incisor may be complicated by lack of space.

Immediate treatment

1. Initially, both parents and child need reassurance and an explanation of the stages of treatment. They should be told that the protective cap is only a temporary measure.
2. No attempt should be made to trim or disc the crown at this stage.
3. A layer of calcium hydroxide paste is applied to the whole of the exposed dentine.
4. Zinc phosphate or polycarboxylate cement is added to form a complete thick layer over the fracture surface.
5. One of the following protective caps is constructed

Fracture T band is welded from soft stainless steel tape (5 mm × 0·15 mm) into a T shape (Fig. 5.8*a*) which is adapted to the fractured crown. The two arms of the T encircle the crown and after removal and welding the band is returned to the tooth where the upright of the T is adapted over the incisal surface, removed, welded and the whole structure carefully trimmed and polished (Fig. 5.8*b*). The occlusion is checked and the band cemented on to the tooth with zinc phosphate cement (Fig. 5.8*c*). Retention of the T band depends upon its fitting as high up on the cervical half of the crown as possible and especially so where the fracture has reduced the crown substance in an unfavourable manner.

The advantages of the fracture T band are that it is strong, clean and retentive.

Preformed steel crowns. Graded sizes are available commercially which only require selection, cervical trimming and adjustment for occlusal height. They are inserted with zinc phosphate cement, but the cutting of a labial window in the steel, sometimes advised to improve the appearance, should be avoided, as this does little to

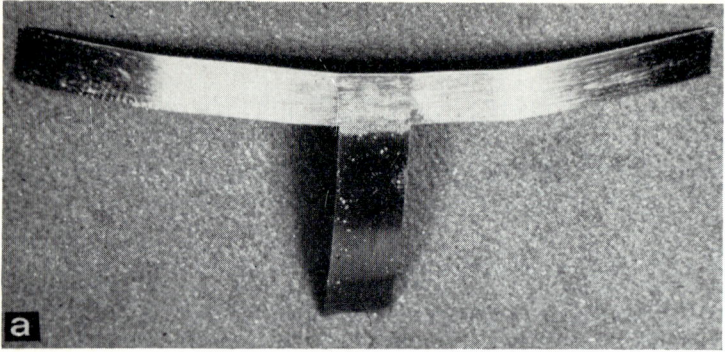

Fig. 5.8*a*, *b*, *c*. Construction of a stainless steel protective band for
fractured incisors.
(*a*) Stainless steel tape welded into a T-form.

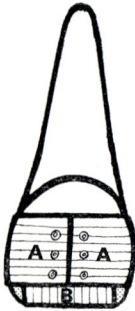

(*b*) Diagram showing arms (A) encircling
the crown, where they are 'pinched' together on the labial surface and secured
with a 'spot' weld. The 'upright' (B) is
adapted over the incisal edge and passed
beneath the band (A). After removal from
the tooth, a series of spot welds shown on
the labial surface converts the band into
a rigid structure.

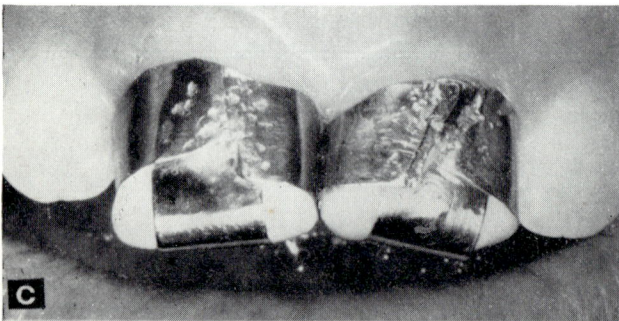

(*c*) Completed fracture bands cemented in position.

improve the aesthetics and severely reduces the effective retention of the crown. It is usually unnecessary and certainly inadvisable to disc away proximal crown tissue from the fractured tooth in order to facilitate the fitting of the preformed crown the purpose of which, after all, is to protect.

Twin silver cap. In circumstances where the plane of the crown fracture is oblique and unfavourable for obtaining adequate band retention (Fig. 5.9*a*) or where two adjacent incisors are similarly

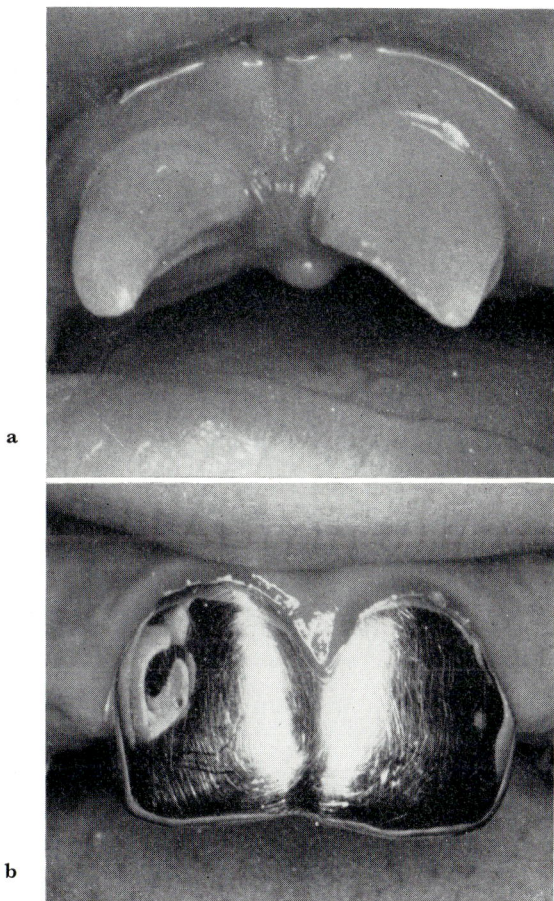

Fig. 5.9*a* and *b*. (*a*) Adjacent fractured central incisors with unfavourable oblique fracture planes.
(*b*) Cast twin silver caps, which obtain retention from reciprocally available crown surfaces.

affected, a cast silver twin cap may be constructed (Fig. 5.9*b*). It is designed to share any remaining proximal surfaces of the two incisors to aid retention and may also be of help as a splinting device if one of the incisors is loose. Its disadvantages are that it is aesthetically poor and it requires an intermediate alginate impression stage before the twin cap can be cast and inserted.

Temporary acrylic crowns. Cellulose acetate crown-forms are available which can be used as a temporary protective device when filled with either zinc oxide/eugenol or with autopolymerising acrylic resin.

No preparation of the tooth is necessary for this temporary measure other than the protective layers to the fractured surface. The acetate crown-form is trimmed cervically; height, and occlusion tested, and a suitable acrylic shade chosen. The crown-form filled with the prepared resin is repositioned on the fractured tooth. Excess is wiped away cervically and then the outer cellulose cover is removed when the crown is set.

ADVANTAGES. 1. Aesthetically a very pleasing result can be obtained and in some cases it may be difficult to improve upon the appearance even when the final acrylic jacket crown is constructed. It has a wide variety of uses as an immediate measure and often helps to allay the emotional trauma experienced by teenage girls who suddenly find that a fall has resulted in an unsightly dental appearance.

2. Its ease of construction makes it a method which can be undertaken without special equipment such as welders.

3. In nearly all circumstances it can be applied without the need to disc or adjust the fractured tooth.

DISADVANTAGES. 1. The fractured plane should always be protected as described because of the irritant nature of the setting autopolymerising resin in the crown-form. Failure to do so may result in pulp injury especially where large areas of dentine are exposed.

2. The temporary acrylic crown is not strong and will deform, wear and loosen under masticatory forces within a short period of time. The weak bonding of the acrylic allows a deformation to occur so that the cap loses its adhesion to the fractured crown surface and falls off.

3. If the loss of crown tissue is extensive or the plane of the fracture is very oblique and unfavourable the remaining tooth substance may not be adequate to retain the temporary acrylic cap. In these circumstances a protective T band offers greater hope of retention.

4. It should be emphasised that this type of protective crown is

entirely temporary and offers no hope as a long-term or even intermediate treatment for the fractured tooth.

Intermediate treatment

After a period of approximately eight weeks the vitality of the injured tooth is assessed (see Chapter 2) and, if satisfactory, a firm restoration with improved appearance is provided for the protected crown. This is still an interim stage to restore the tooth until recovery has occurred and the eruption has reached a satisfactory level. The kind of restoration needed is one which requires only the minimal removal of crown tissue to obtain effective retention. Four types are suitable at this stage:

> Basket crown
> Pinlays
> Shoulderless jacket crown
> Staple restoration

Basket crown. The restoration is so named because it carries a fine cervical band of gold (the basket handle) to increase retention.

PREPARATION. Using a disc-guard, the crown is sliced mesially and distally and the incisal 1 mm removed (Fig. 5.10*a*, *b*, *c*, *d*, *e*). There is usually a slight cervical undercut on the labial aspect of upper incisors and this should be removed sufficiently to allow the thin labial extension of gold to seat as far up the crown as possible. The removal of a thin layer of palatal enamel is necessary to allow for the thin palatal veneer of gold. Where the crown is extensively fractured and retention is at a premium, a palatal pin may be added. The basket crown wax pattern must be constructed indirectly and a rubber base impression will be required. A preliminary alginate impression is used for the construction of a special tray. Models are cast and the pattern is carved with a window so that a facing can be added when the gold restoration is cemented in place. If there is considerable loss of crown tissue a better appearance is obtained by removing a thin slice of labial enamel so that the whole labial surface can be restored with acrylic resin which is cured on to the finished gold restoration (Fig. 5.11). The aesthetics are usually superior to those obtained when autopolymerising resin is brushed on as a facing.

The wax pattern is carved in such a way that the cervical bar is left broad at this stage and reduced during the trimming and polishing stages of the cast gold. Two sprues are used—one from the incisal edge and the other from the centre of the cervical bar

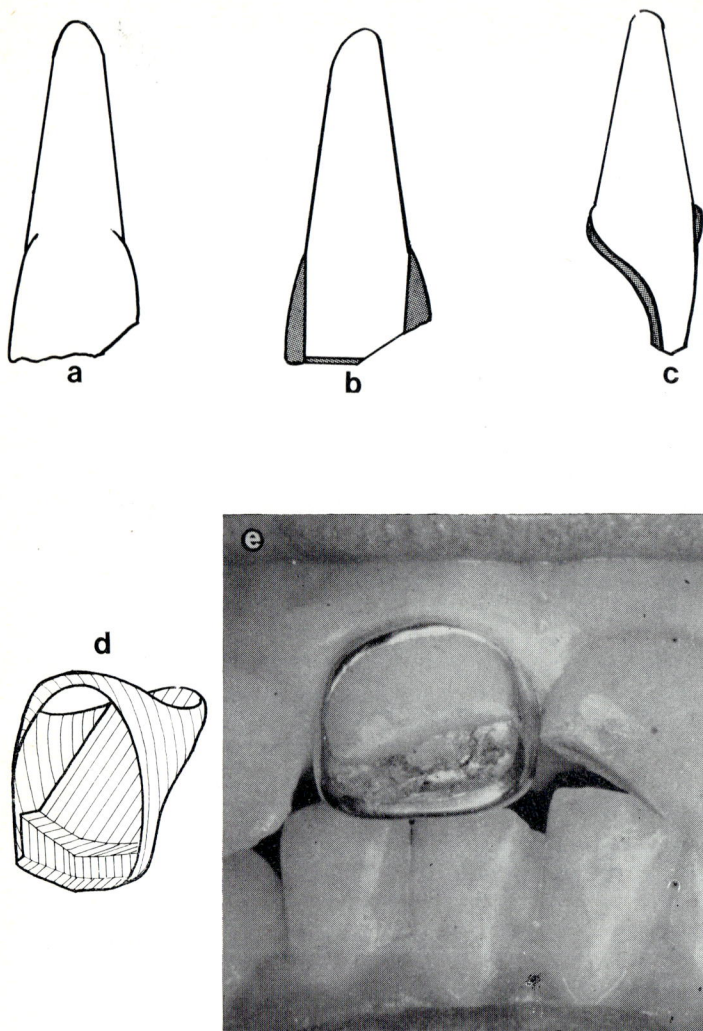

Fig. 5.10a, b, c, d, e. Stages of basket crown preparation.

(a) Fractured incisor.

(b) Reduction of proximal tissue and straightening of ragged incisal edge.

(c) Removal of palatal enamel and labial cervical undercut.

(d) Diagram of the pattern illustrating the fitting surfaces of the basket crown.

(e) Photograph of crown cemented in position 1/ and awaiting the addition of facing.

and the pattern is invested and cast in 18-carat gold. Adequate temporary crowns are constructed to prevent adjacent and opposing incisors moving into the space provided by the crown perparation.

Pinlays and pinledges. The value of pinlay restorations is that they give a retentive restoration with minimum disturbance of tooth tissue during preparation. However, there are certain limitations to their use based on the fact that the greater the degree of crown loss, the greater the number of pins, the deeper and the more difficult

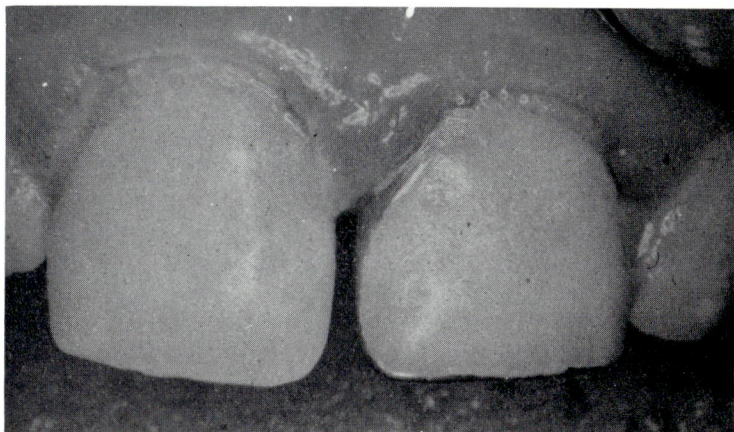

Fig. 5.11. Intermediate restoration of /1 by means of a cast gold shell crown on to which has been processed a standard acrylic facing.

it is to position them in the remaining tooth substance if the pulp is to remain uninjured. A situation arises, when in the incisor with a completely formed apex, it is more expeditious and more aesthetic to devitalise and root fill the tooth and construct a post crown. Pinlay construction is therefore normally confined in young fractured incisors to the replacement of incisal tip or edge, although the method can be modified for use on an extensively fractured crown for which a partial pulp amputation (pulpotomy) has been carried out.

The pinlay is designed so that its intracoronal retention by means of pins should resist displacing forces acting upon it during mastication. At the same time, however, the pinholes must be positioned so that they are kept within the safety margins and will not injure the pulp (Fig. 5.12).

Loss of incisal tip. Where a mesial or distal tip of an incisor is lost, the pinlay preparation should include a principal pinhole sited just inside the junction of dentine with enamel where the fracture plane reaches the proximal surface. The depth of the pin should be 2-3 mm and parallel to the long axis of the tooth. The enamel edge is straightened and a slight bevel is introduced to the palatal aspect of the fractured plane. A second minor pinhole is cut in the mid-incisal position not deeper than 1 mm. The diameter of both pinholes is the same as a No. $\frac{1}{2}$ round, rose-head bur.

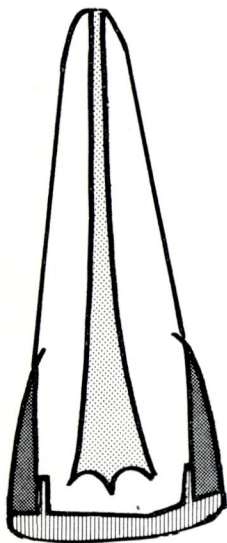

FIG. 5.12. Diagram illustrating the safety positions for pins in pinlay preparation.

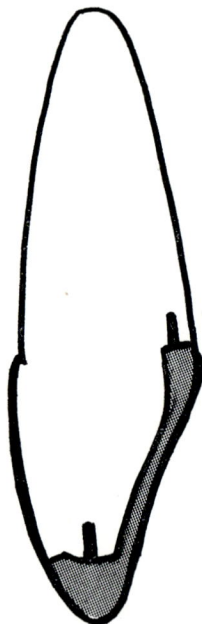

FIG. 5.13. Diagram showing location of an additional pin which is carried on the palatal veneer at the cervical margin.

This type of restoration is only suitable for the loss of a relatively small portion of the crown, and it will be appreciated that when the whole incisal third of the crown has become involved the intra-coronal retention must be increased by the addition of a further pin at the level of the palatal cervical margin (Fig 5.13) and modification of the shallow pinhole into a more substantial retention. It is usually necessary to remove a thin layer of palatal enamel so that a gold veneer can extend to cover the pin head at the cervical margin.

The pinholes are made using precision cutters and the appropriate plastic pins adjusted to the depth of the hole so that the head is clear and will allow the indirect impression material to surround it.

Parallelism between pins is necessary if they are to fit their respective holes accurately. Where only one principal pin is used in the replacement of a small tip and combined with a smaller minor pin, parallelism presents no problem and can be done free-hand. However, three-pin preparations require the use of a paralleling device. A special tray is required for an impression using rubber base but before so doing the plastic pins are placed *in situ* with 2 mm of their heads projecting from their pinholes. When the impression is removed with the pin heads enclosed within it, each pin shaft is given a coat of glycerine before the model is cast. Later a wax squash bite and lower alginate impression are recorded, the pinholes filled with wax and a temporary crown or band fitted to the incisor. When the impression is removed from the model, a fresh pin is inserted in each pinhole so that the head can be enclosed in the indirect inlay wax pattern and an appropriate window cut for a facing where necessary. Investment and casting take place in the usual manner, 18-carat gold being used.

Very small variations in the parallelism of the pins preventing the final seating of the restoration can be overcome by slightly widening the pinholes which will allow the pins to ease into position. However it is essential in all cases that the pinholes be filled with fresh zinc phosphate cement as the restoration is finally seated. The windows previously prepared in the gold are lined with an opacifying agent to mask the appearance of the metal before the autopoly-merising resin is added.

'Shoulderless' jacket crowns. Preparation consists of discing the tooth so that all the axial crown surfaces converge incisally. Relatively little tissue is removed from the crown and there is minimal disturbance of the pulp. It is a particularly useful intermediate restoration for young incisors which are discoloured or unsightly as a result of injury, caries or hypoplasia. Any remaining incisal edge is reduced by 2 mm (Fig. 5.14) and the minimum of labial and palatal enamel removed with a diamond wheel so that there are no undercut areas and the contact with the lower incisors is cleared. Before completing the final stage in the preparation there are two main problems to be considered with this type of intermediate restoration and the most important one is the finish of the crown at the cervical margin. Since the crown is intended to last for a number of years until a traditional jacket crown can be prepared, it is essential that the neck of the considered crown should not allow gingival stagnation. 'Knife-edge finishes' can be satisfactorily constructed in gold, but in acrylic resin this finish is both unaesthetic and unhealthy. The word 'shoulderless', should therefore be interpreted as a minimum cervical preparation so that there may be a narrow ledge for direct abutment of the acrylic at the neck of the tooth.

The second problem relates to the fact that only a small amount of the original crown was removed and as a result the jacket if con-

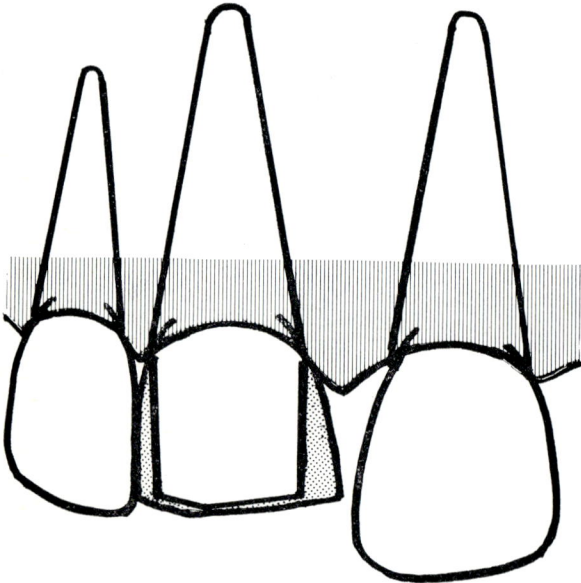

FIG. 5.14. Diagram illustrating the minimal preparation required for the construction of a shoulderless jacket crown.

structed to the same size will be thin and weak. The only way to maintain a strong jacket crown is to increase its bulk. Providing the crown length matches adjacent teeth and the cervical trim is neat, a moderate increase in thickness is well tolerated.

There are cases, however, where incisor crown space is at a premium and where crowding and unfavourable Class II division 2 incisor relationships will not allow larger crown substitutes. In these circumstances a gold thimble crown with complete labial facing is preferable. The final stage is the preparation of the minimal shoulder, which is cut to a depth of 1·0 mm before the rest of the enamel is disced. Since most severe crown fractures result in great reduction of retention all walls of the preparation should be kept as parallel as possible in an axial plane.

The impression is recorded with rubber base material, a cement model cast and the crown built up and processed in the normal way after trimming slightly the cervical margins of the model. In some circumstances it is preferable to use the face of a stock acrylic tooth and re-wax the back and neck to fit the model. It is essential to

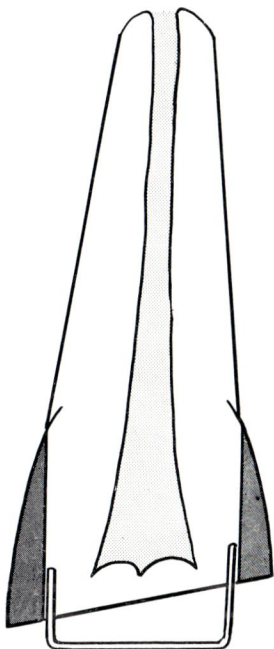

FIG. 5.15. Diagram of a semi-permanent restoration using a stainless steel staple shown cemented in position.

remember to fit a temporary crown after preparation has been finished; otherwise alteration in the occlusal and proximal relations of the affected tooth will make it impossible to fit the crown later.

Staple restorations. This type of restoration uses a stainless steel staple constructed so that each end is cemented into prepared holes on the fractured crown in order to retain a plastic tip. Preparation is simple and consists of cutting with a No. $\frac{1}{2}$ round rose-head bur a principal pinhole 2 mm deep at the enamel/dentine junction interproximally. A second stabilising pinhole is cut 2 mm in dentine at the incisal edge. Soft 0·2 mm stainless steel wire is roughened with a stone and bent into an arc between the two holes and cemented in position (Fig. 5.15). When the sensitive dentine area has been protected with a layer of zinc phosphate cement the tip of a celluloid crown-form is cut to shape as a matrix, filled with selected silicate cement and placed on the tooth. Trimming and polishing are finished at a later stage.

MINIMAL ADJUSTMENTS TO INCISAL EDGE. It is not always necessary to restore the fractured tip of the incisor to its full crown length. In some cases when fracture of 1/1 has involved enamel only on one incisor but where the adjacent tooth needs a substantial restoration,

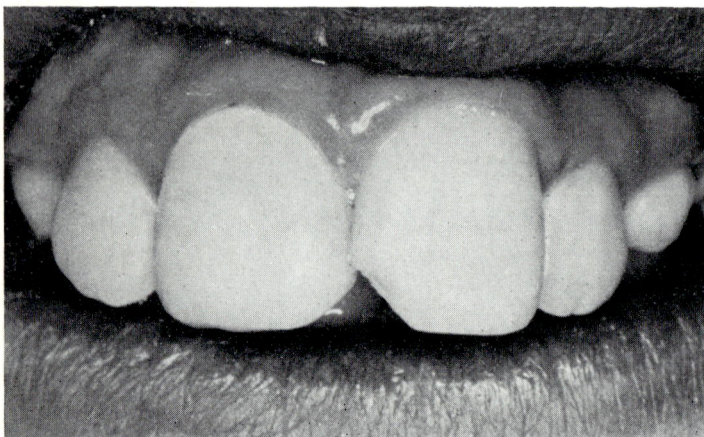

FIG. 5.16. The 1/ crown has been extensively injured by trauma and replaced by a jacket crown. The fracture of /1 has involved the mesial tip and a minimal amount of the incisal edge. The edge has been straightened and the adjacent jacket crown adjusted to balance this appearance.

for example by jacket crown of pinledge, it can be restored short of its original crown length. If this course is adopted the slight fracture irregularity of the corresponding tooth will only need carefully discing to produce an acceptable level (Fig. 5.16).

Fractures of crown involving pulp

Whilst it is true to say that all fractures bring about a reaction in the pulp as a result of increased thermal and chemical stimuli, this section deals with direct traumatic pulp exposures (see Fig. 2.7). When this type of fracture occurs, endodontic therapy will be necessary and depends on clinical and radiographic appreciation of the factors already discussed. If there are no contraindictions then treatment will be based upon pulp size and apex development. vitality and the prognosis for restoring the tooth.

At approximately ten and a half years of age the apices of 1/1 are completed and the canals sufficiently reduced in diameter to allow root-fillings to be inserted if necessary. If the fracture exposing the pulp occurs earlier in the development of the teeth, the operator has to contend with the wide, funnel-shaped apex which offers additional endodontic problems, not the least of which is the short root. It becomes a matter of some importance therefore to use techniques

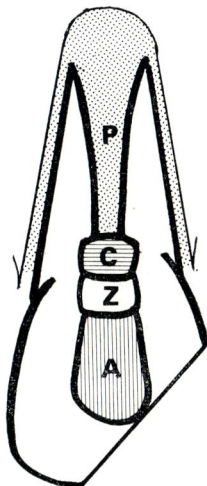

FIG. 5.17. Diagram of pulpotomy preparation and dressing layers.
Key: P = Pulp
C = Calcium hydroxide
Z = Zinc phosphate cement
A = Amalgam

which will allow root growth to proceed normally by encouraging a localised healing of the pulp. The operation performed on the exposed pulp of an immature incisor is called a *pulpotomy* or *partial pulpectomy*. It consists of amputating, under local anaesthesia, the whole of the coronal pulp tissue and placing a thick calcium hydroxide layer directly on to this surface, which is then capped with zinc phosphate cement and amalgam (Fig. 5.17).

What are the advantages of pulpotomy?   1. Pulpotomy removes the infected ulcer at the exposure site.

2. By cutting back the pulp tissue within the rigid crown structure healing can take place undisturbed under the various therapeutic layers. In other words the new amputation surface is deeply recessed within the surrounding structures and this promotes healing and freedom from pain.

3. The operation allows the apex to complete, and if a post crown is eventually needed to restore the tooth, the fully developed internal and periapical structures together with adequate root length permit routine endodontic preparations.

4. It is a simple operation with an 80 per cent success rate.

The healing process at the amputation site is unusual and depends upon the alkaline pH of the calcium hydroxide which brings about an intensive localised superficial necrosis where the pulp is in contact with it. The deeper layers of the pulp appear to be undamaged in the successful pulpotomy during the healing process although degenerative changes may sometimes occur later. The alkaline

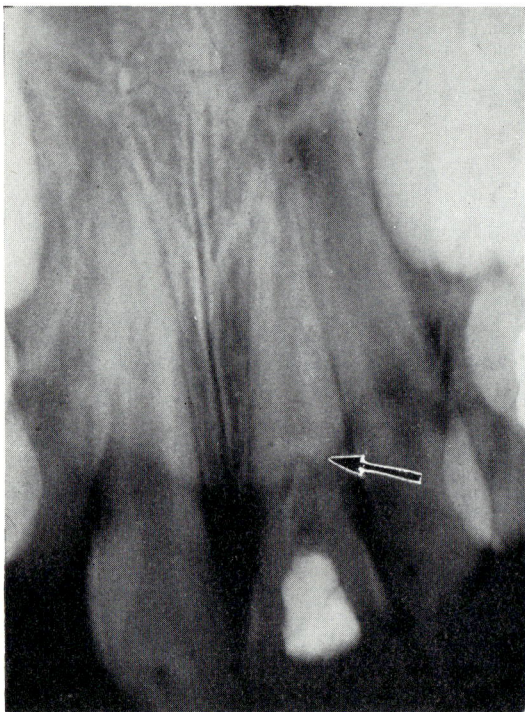

FIG. 5.18. Radiograph showing calcific bridge (arrow) at the site of pulp amputation.

calcium hydroxide destroys nerve fibres at the amputation site, and also reduces bacterial contamination in the area. Its effects are limited to the area immediately adjacent to the contact zone, and no deeper hyperaemia occurs so that normal pulp circulation can continue. The chronic round cell infiltration experienced when zinc oxide/eugenol and other materials are used, does not occur with calcium hydroxide. When the superficial necrosis is complete, calcific changes occur in the pulpal tissues immediately below this layer. (Fig. 5.18). The calcium ions for this reaction are not taken from the calcium hydroxide but are part of the normal pulp fluid exchange system and the calcific bridge builds up to a layer of approximately 1 mm. Variations in thickness can be observed and occasionally a breach may be seen in the layer where a pulp remnant has been incompletely removed and has led to a failure in sealing off the pulp, resulting in its subsequent necrosis.

Pulpotomy technique. 1. Apply aqueous Hibitane (0·05 per cent) to the labial sulcus and teeth associated with the traumatised area.

2. Surface anaesthetic is applied.

3. One millilitre of a local anaesthetic is injected into the labial sulcus over the apex of the affected tooth. Where anaesthesia is difficult to obtain a second injection should be given (0·5 ml) into the interdental papilla distal to the tooth. A palatal injection is usually unnecessary. In the lower arch, 1 ml is given into the labial sulcus and half a cartridge injected lingually after three minutes. The criteria of success for the pulpotomy depends on whether the pulp can be maintained in a vital state sufficiently long for the root to complete its normal development.

4. Anaesthesia at the pulp exposure site is tested by gently moving a probe point across the area to detect sensation.

5. The tooth is isolated with cotton rolls and saliva ejector or with rubber dam.

6. A sterile endodontic kit containing reamers, broaches, burs and necessary hand instruments is placed in readiness. The initial opening into the pulp chamber should be through the lingual fossa, irrespective of the traumatic injury site. The two important reasons for this approach are that good vision and access are essential for a successful pulpotomy and the unnecessary destruction of crown tissue takes place if an exposed pulp-horn has to be widened and extended to allow removal of the remaining coronal pulp. High-speed airotor diamonds are used to establish a 3 mm entry through the cingulum. Just before the breach into the pulp is made, the access is swabbed with Hibitane (0·05 per cent) and the engine changed to slow speed with a No. 3 rose-head bur which is again replaced by a No. 8 rose-head bur to increase the access. The pulp tissue is slowly cut back until the whole of the coronal pulp is removed. It is preferable to amputate the pulp tissue with a rose-head bur rather than with an excavator, since the latter tends to leave strands of pulp tissue attached and difficult to detect. Care should be taken so that all small remnants of the pulp-horns have been removed, since these will tend to discolour the crown due to subsequent decomposition.

7. The crown chamber is washed out with sterile saline, and a calcium hydroxide powder or paste inserted over the amputation site and left for two minutes. As the superficial necrosis begins at the amputation site the bleeding will stop and the cavity is again washed to clear away the paste and remaining clot so that an effective inspection can be carried out. If blood clot is allowed to remain crown discoloration will again occur due to decomposition.

8. A thick layer of calcium hydroxide paste is inserted over the amputation site followed by a layer of zinc phosphate cement sealed with an amalgam or a silicate filling.

9. A temporary cap should be placed over the tooth to maintain its spatial relations within the arch and six-monthly radiographs are taken to determine the progress of the tooth and evidence of calcific bridge formation.

Where there is extensive fracture of the crown exposing the pulp, pulpotomy is still the method of choice, but the real problem comes when deciding how to restore such a meagre remnant of a crown. Although the long-term plan will be to construct a post crown, the intermediate stage must be a compromise. The pulp is therefore amputated to a higher level in the canal and in this way a short wide post can be combined with a single palatal pin in a gold backing with diaphragm and collar (Fig. 5.19). It is essential, however, to keep the crown length as short as possible so that there is less tendency for the crown to be displaced during mastication.

Treatment of immature incisors with dead pulps

When one considers the large fluid volume exchange that occurs within the immature pulp, the freedom of circulation via the funnel-shaped apex and the ability of young tissue to recover from injury, it is not surprising that pulp necrosis following trauma is not common. When it does occur, however, the root canal anatomy is such that it is mechanically impossible to fit a rigid root filling through a narrower canal into a broader apical third.

The following procedure is adopted in this situation:

1. Give local infiltration anaesthesia and isolate the tooth as already described.

2. Obtain wide access via the lingual fossa.

3. Remove necrotic pulp tissue taking care not to pass barbed broach into apical tissues.

4. Syringe canal with large volume of sodium hypochlorite solution.

5. Although the canal is too wide for reamers the walls should be

smoothed with large canal files again taking great care not to disturb the periapical tissues. Radiographs of diagnostic reamers are taken.

6. Repeat syringing of canal with normal saline.

7. Using sterile paper points, dry the canal and smear the walls with p-monochlorphenol, sealing in the dressing with cotton wool pledgets and quick-set zinc oxide/eugenol.

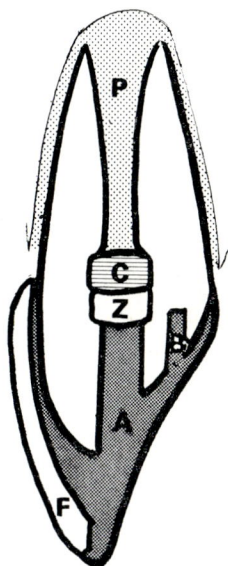

FIG. 5.19. Diagram illustrating the restoration of an incisor following a pulpotomy, where a crown is constructed with a short post into the canal (A) combined with an additional palatal pin (B), and acrylic facing (F).

Key: P = Pulp
C = Calcium hydroxide
Z = Zinc phosphate cement

8. The patient is seen after four days and the canal reamed and dressings repeated using rubber dam to avoid oral contamination.

9. On the third visit the canal should be free from pus and ready to fill. The root filling consists of two layers:

(i) A paste of calcium hydroxide and iodoform (equal parts) is inserted in the apical third with a lentulo canal-filler or alternatively through a syringe. (Proprietory brands are available, e.g. Kri paste).

(ii) A thick gutta-percha roll sufficiently large to fit the wide canal, is prepared by warming a piece of gutta-percha and rolling it to the required thickness between two sterile glass slabs. Its end is cut square and it requires testing in the canal with radiographic control to ensure it has the correct diameter.

When the tooth has been isolated and the calcium hydroxide paste inserted, the gutta-percha filling is used as a plunger to condense the paste into the apical part of the canal. Final adjustment to the position of the gutta-percha can be made after a periapical film has been taken.

10. The coronal access to the canal is sealed with amalgam. (Fig. 5.20).

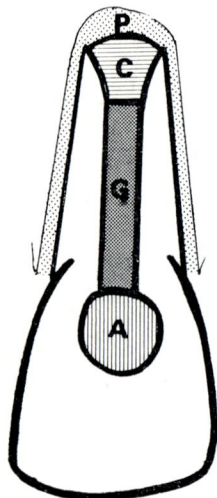

Fig. 5.20. Diagram of root filling for the immature incisor canal.
Key: P = Periodontal ligaments
C = Calcium hydroxide paste
G = Gutta percha filling
A = Amalgam seal

Problem of bacteriological sampling

The second International Conference on Endontics reported in a 1958 consensus that there was no valid evidence to infer that cases with culture control showed any better results than those without such control.

Reports since this time have done little to change the situation except that the healing in the periapical tissues may be slightly accelerated in cases which gave negative cultures before root filling.

What information does bacteriological control give the operator? It has been suggested that it offers the advantage of assessing the bacteriological status of the tooth, and the efficiency of the cleansing technique whilst a persistently positive culture might suggest that other factors such as an accessory root canal might be responsible. A negative culture does not always indicate a bacteria-free canal and, on the other hand, knowing the particular type of organism present in a positive culture rarely causes alteration of the antiseptic medication unless polyantibiotic mixtures are used after testing for sensitivity. There can be little doubt that the importance of correct bio-mechanical preparation cannot be overstressed and is likely to be a much more important factor in the success of the endodontics than the knowledge given by bacteriological sampling.

Root canal medicaments

There was little to show that any advantage could be obtained by using canal antibiotics as compared with antiseptics. Added to this the operator should always be concerned with the risk of developing resistant strains of bacteria where inadequate strengths of the antibiotic were released into the apical tissues by seepage. Hypersensitivity is another factor which has to be considered and adds to the general evidence suggesting that antibiotics used in this situation carry some risk to the patient. On the whole, they are not warranted when other equally effective means are available, e.g. camphorated p-monochlorphenol.

Healing in the open apex

There are a number of cases where, once the root filling described above has been inserted, further apical growth appears possible. To what degree the wide apical funnel is capable of encouraging a partial revascularisation, it is difficult to say, but judging by the radiographic appearance the apex reflects the temporary disturbance in root growth.

Fracture of the root

Fracture of the root, although a relatively uncommon feature in primary incisors, is more frequently met with in the permanent dentition. Its presence may be detected only by chance, or on radiographic investigation of other factors, and this is especially so since the tooth may remain almost symptomless except for slight loosening.

It has already been pointed out that a short sharp blow from a hard object such as a stone is likely to fracture the crown whereas a slower blow from a softer and heavier object, for example a boot, will cause displacement of the tooth as a whole. The type of trauma which could cause root fracture is probably somewhere between these two and is likely to be more frequent where there is a greater root length, i.e. with completed apex.

The position of the root fracture affects the prognosis for the tooth. Where it is of a vertical or oblique variety involving the crown, there can be no real hope of delaying extraction of the tooth. On the

F

other hand fractures near the apex have a much better outlook, partly because the crown is still firmly supported by the major root portion and also since, if loss of pulp vitality occurs there are good prospects for resection of the small apical fragment. It is an interesting feature of fractures in the apical one-third that these often show little displacement of the two fractured root ends except where an abscess has supervened. Whether the level at which the fracture occurs on the root is a reflection of the force of the injury is not known nor is it possible to say whether the greater displacement of the root ends, often observed in mid-root fractures, is a reflection of the force of the blow or of subsequent movement of the coronal fragment with its seriously reduced attachment.

Healing can occur between fractured root ends without any loss of function or of pulp vitality. It is likely that this takes place in many cases completely unknown to the patient and operator alike, considering the number of untreated traumatic injuries that must occur. The reunion of the parts may be calcific, although where this occurs it is almost impossible to detect, but a fibrous band may join the two ends in a good functional relationship but with slightly increased mobility.

Treatment. The immediate treatment for all root fractures, with the exception of those affecting the crown, should be splinting, without any attempt at pulp treatment in the early stages. Immobilisation allows healing to occur in the torn periodontal fibres and also reduces the risk of infection entering by this route from the damaged gingival crevice. Fixation of the fractured root encourages healing by calcific or fibrous means and reduces embarrassment to the pulp. In all forms of early treatment great care should be taken not to displace the crown fragment because this may cause additional injury to the pulp.

SPLINTS. The most satisfactory splintage for an incisor with a fractured root is a cast metal splint. It is important to avoid wire ligation or orthodontic band splints since small amounts of torque introduced during fitting and adjusting these materials will alter the optimal relations of the fractured ends. Splinting coverage for one or two upper incisors with root fractures should extend to include 3/3. Since tilting of the fractured teeth is to be avoided during the impression stage a small lower tray is prepared by adding post dam wax behind 3/3 area to confine the alginate to the relevant site. The teeth are coated with glycerine to allow easy removal of the impression with minimum disturbance of the affected teeth. A wax squash bite is inadvisable for these cases since it may cause additional injury to the fractured teeth and is unnecessary since the splint will inevitably produce a temporary alteration in the incisal occlusion due to the thickness of the material covering the teeth.

When the models are produced, undercuts around the teeth are blocked out and the relevant teeth foiled, waxed up, invested and the splint cast in silver (Fig. 5.21). It is advisable to make a small

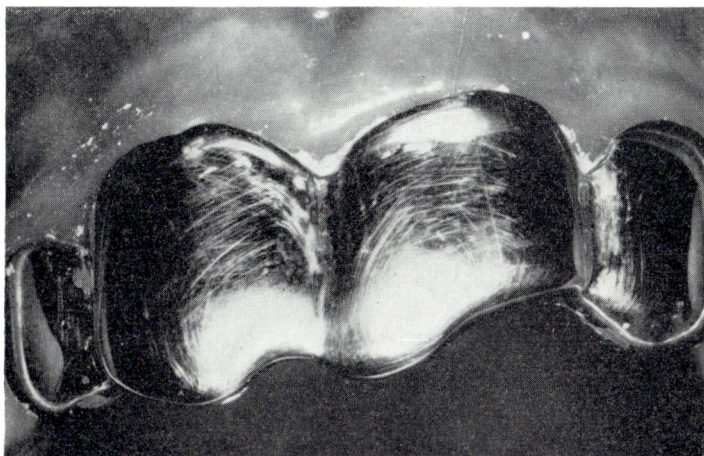

FIG. 5.21. Cast silver splint for 21/12

perforation in the silver where it covers the lingual fossa of the affected incisor since this provides a rapid entry port if endodontic therapy becomes necessary without the need to remove the splint, and will allow the easy seating of the splint whilst it is being cemented.

Although, because of its rigidity and strength, the most effective splints are made of silver, processed acrylic splints can be manufactured. They require a greater bulk of material to be effectively rigid and where retention is poor they may need extending to cover all the teeth in the arch. Aesthetically tooth-coloured acrylic is superior to silver and this may be a factor of considerable importance for a patient who is wearing a splint for eight to twelve weeks. When the splint has been manufactured it is tested in the mouth before cementation with zinc phosphate cement.

In midroot and apical third fractures the splint is left in position for eight to twelve weeks after which it is first cut away from the injured tooth and removed. Providing that the vitality responses are normal and periapical radiographs show no evidence of periodontal disturbance then the tooth should be kept under review. If, however, the tooth becomes non-vital, apical root resection can be carried out after first root filling the canal as far as the fractured plane, twenty-four hours before hand.

APICECTOMY TECHNIQUE. Preparation of the patient before hand should include a warning of the possibility of postoperative swelling and an antibiotic cover should be prescribed even for routine cases. Any root fillings are usually completed at a previous appointment but may be carried out at the time of apicectomy.

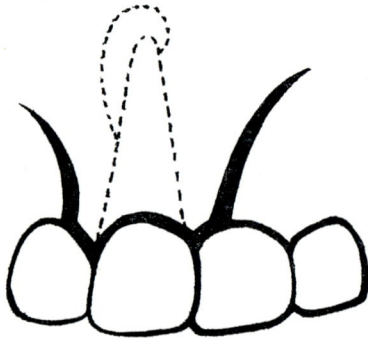

FIG. 5.22. Diagram illustrating an extended incision to give good access when lateral periodontal bone is involved in the apical root resection.

1. Infiltration anaesthesia is given in the following form: 2 ml solution over the tooth involved, 1 ml over each adjacent tooth, and if 21/12 are involved, 0·5 ml slowly into the naso-palatine canal.

2. A semilunar incision is made and the flap reflected. Alternatively, where the periapical lesion is seen on the radiograph to extend along the lateral aspect of the root, an incision into the gingival sulcus (Fig. 5.22) will give better access to the pathological area.

3. The periapical plate of bone is removed with a No. 10 rose-head bur to expose the apex, but great care must be taken to avoid disturbing roots of adjacent teeth.

4. The removal of the apical fragment is carried out so that the fissure bur cuts through the root at an oblique angle which will give direct access for a retrograde amalgam filling. The remaining root end is prepared with an apical cavity using a small rose-head bur and a retrograde amalgam filling inserted (Fig. 5.23). The retrograde amalgam is a useful apical seal especially where a previously inserted root filling is inadequate. However, care must be taken to

clear away blood and other debris before the amalgam is inserted and also to ensure that any metal filling fragments are removed from the bone cavity.

5. The bone cavity is syringed with sterile saline and a final inspection carried out before the flap is closed with about three 3/O or 4/O black silk sutures.

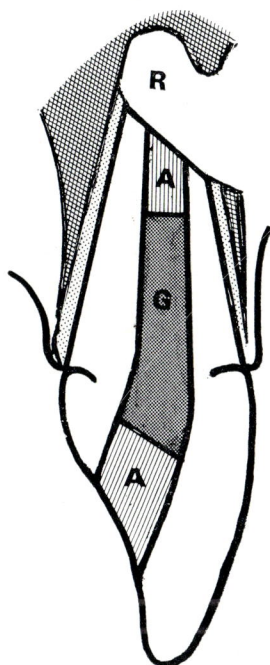

Fig. 5.23. Diagram of a lateral view of an upper incisor with a resected apex showing the oblique angle of the cut which allows easier access for packing the apical amalgam (A).
Key: R = Resected apex cavity
A = Amalgam
G = Gutta percha

6. Postoperatively the patient is given soluble aspirin tablets and the sutures are removed seven to ten days later. The teeth are periodically reviewed with radiographs which should show evidence of bone reformation by the end of twelve months. A splint may be necessary if the tooth is loose following removal of a large apical fragment.

Apicectomy is indicated in a number of endodontic situations which include:

(*a*) Apical root fractures, deformed or abnormally developed apices and accessory apical canals.
(*b*) Broken reamers and files in canal.
(*c*) Chronic apical granuloma which may occur as a result of

pulp necrosis, chronic pulp infection, or unsuccessful endodontic therapy, and overspill of root filling into periapical spaces.

(d) It may be used to ensure affective periapical seal by retrograde root fillings.

Apicectomy is contraindicated during an acute inflammatory phase or where there is close proximity to the inferior dental neurovascular bundle, poor access or visibility or where the roots protrude significantly into the maxillary antrum.

Subluxated and luxated teeth

The type of blow which results in displacement of the tooth has been discussed. Mobility is a dominant feature and in certain cases the tooth is pushed into a position where it interferes with normal centric occlusion. Sometimes several teeth are displaced as a group and fractures of the alveolar bone may be associated with this type of injury. When complete dislodgement (luxation) of the whole tooth occurs the operator is involved with biomechanical problems of retention and reattachment of the disrupted periodontal tissues.

Pulp vitality is the principal problem with subluxated incisors even though many periodontal fibres are torn during the movement of the tooth, reattachment and healing is usually straightforward providing the tooth can be splinted into a good occlusal relationship.

If an upper incisor has been forced back by the blow into a lingual relationship it should be moved gently back into its original position and splinted. There is a recognised danger that in so doing any remaining vital periapical neurovascular tissue may be severed, but it is generally found that few of these can survive extremes of traumatic movement. If, on the other hand, the tooth is left in a maloccluded position, the abnormal bite may cause further damage to the periapical tissues and possibly root resorption.

Treatment for displaced incisors. 1. Routine and other investigations are outlined in Chapter 2.

2. If a tooth is displaced or very mobile it should be gently realigned within the arch and an alginate impression recorded for construction of a cast silver or an acrylic splint.

3. A temporary foil splint is constructed to immobilise the injured teeth. It may be made of cooking-foil or any similar adaptable metal from which a curved strip $1\frac{1}{2} \times 1$ inch is moulded and trimmed on any suitable dental model. The splint is extended to include two adjacent teeth either side of the injured units and trimmed peripherally to rest on the gingival tissues (Fig. 5.24). After cleansing

in alcohol the splint is tried in the mouth for final adaptation and after drying the teeth, it is cemented with copper cement and left in position whilst a more functional splint is being manufactured.

4. The cast or processed splint carries a perforation over the palatal aspect of the affected tooth in case urgent endodontic access is required once the splint is in position.

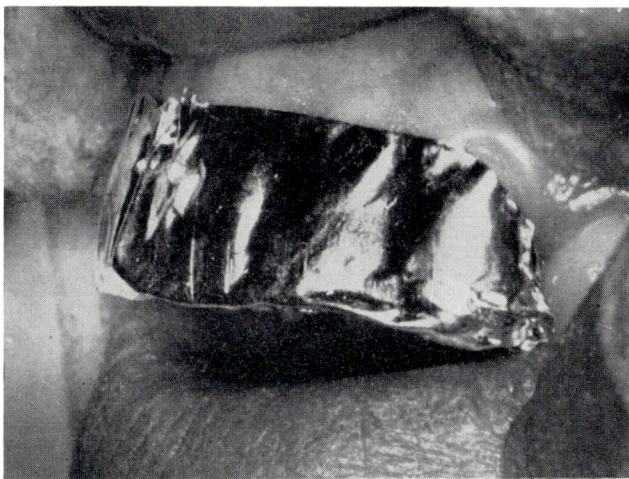

Fig. 5.24. Lateral view of a temporary foil splint cemented over 321/123

The splint should be left in position for approximately eight weeks when the tooth is again radiographed. Occasionally even minor traumatic episodes give rise to pulp calcification, which is a histochemical process probably associated with alteration in the vascular supply. It seldom occurs in immature incisors which are richly supplied with blood vessels.

Dislodged incisors (luxated incisors). When the tooth has been dislodged from its socket the operator has three problems which he must consider.

1. Replantation. Preparing and splinting the tooth firmly in place.
2. Prophylactic antitetanic therapy and antibiotics.
3. Prognosis.

1. TOOTH PREPARATION AND SPLINTING. Reattachment between root cementum and socket is more likely to occur if the tooth has been only recently dislodged and if it has been kept moist but

uncontaminated by chemicals especially antiseptics. It must be capable of being replanted and splinted firmly in its original position.

Technique. The crown of the dislodged tooth is grasped firmly in a damp napkin and the root gently washed in sterile saline. The apex is resected and the pulp removed from the apical end. Once the

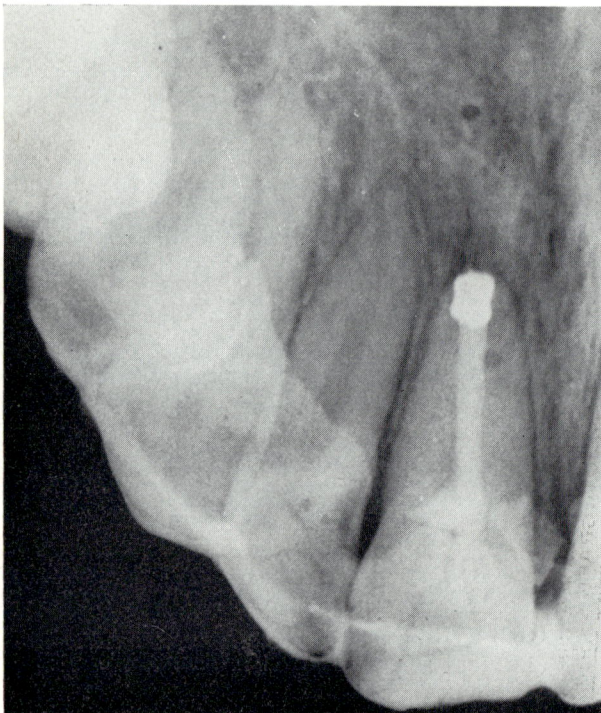

FIG. 5.25. Radiograph of a replanted central incisor showing root resection, filling and apical amalgam seal. The tooth is held firm by a temporary foil splint.

canal is reamed and the fragments syringed away, a suitable gutta-percha point is covered with a thin mix of zinc oxide eugenol paste and packed into the canal, being finally sealed in with a retrograde amalgam.

The clot is removed from the socket, the tooth repositioned (Fig. 5.25) and splinted in place with a temporary foil splint described above. This can be left for two weeks after which it is carefully cut away from the tooth and impressions recorded for a cast silver or acrylic splint which is to be used for a further eight weeks.

2. PROTECTION AGAINST TETANUS AND OTHER INFECTIONS. The risk of tetanus is a serious one where the injury is deep or where there is gross soft tissue damage and especially if it has occurred over land grazed by ruminants or on garden soils prepared with natural manures. The patient should be referred to his medical practitioner or hospital outpatients department for advice. The child may only

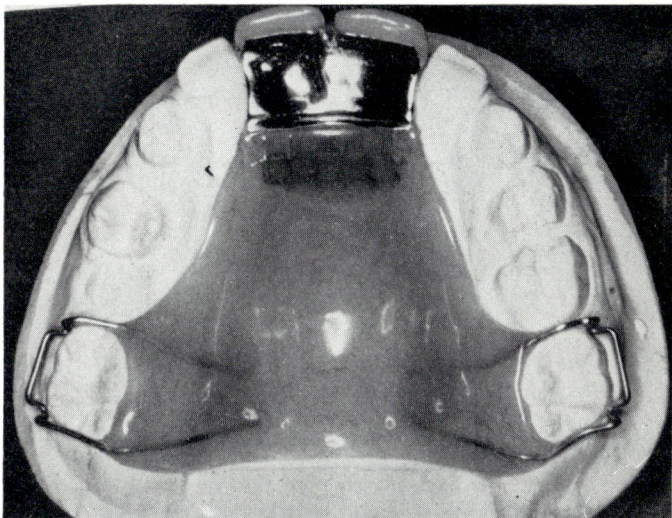

Fig. 5.26. Prosthetic replacement for lost incisors, using Adam's cribs on 6/6 to increase the retention.

require a booster dose of tetanus toxoid if he has previously received protection, but in any case antibiotics by mouth should always be prescribed in these types of injury:

Phenoxymethylpenicillin every 6 hours.
    62·5 mg for infants.
    125 mg under 10 years.
    250 mg over 10 years.

3. PROGNOSIS. Although cases are known where replanted teeth continue to be retained indefinitely, the majority become absorbed by the end of five years. The reasons why such a successful reattachment should be followed by resorptive processes at the root surface are not known.

Prosthetic replacements of lost incisors. Upper and lower alginate impressions are recorded together with a wax squash bite and a selected tooth shade. The design of the partial denture should be such that in the first instance it uses Adam's cribs to aid its retention (Fig. 5.26) These are constructed so that they engage the buccal undercuts on the upper cheek teeth in manner similar to that used for removable orthodontic appliances. By means of this retention it is possible to reduce the remainder of the plate to a shape which avoids contact and stagnation against other teeth except in the replacement and crib attachment areas.

When the patient has become accustomed to wearing a partial denture, subsequent replacements can take the form of a spoon without the use of cribs. All acrylic dentures should be processed in radio-opaque materials which may be detected radiographically in case they are subsequently fractured or swallowed during injury.

6   Dental Care of Handicapped Children

It is difficult to obtain an accurate assessment of the number of mentally and physically handicapped children in Britain. Estimates place the number at more than 80,000 physically handicapped children who were receiving education outside ordinary schools in 1965 and that a further 22,000 who were educationally subnormal or maladjusted were awaiting entry to special schools.

Many dental surgeons are finding that as they accept their full share in community responsibility, a greater number of handicapped children are coming under their care. It is recognised that the handicap may not be confined to physical deformity or mental subnormality, but there is an increasing awareness of the challenge offered by maladjusted and emotionally inadequate children. They require special consideration in planning and treatment in the same way as the children suffering from cardiac disease or haemophilia need specific precautions for their handicap.

Table 6.1 indicates the proportion of major groups of physical handicap in children attending special day and boarding schools in England and Wales.

TABLE 6.1

Disability	Percentage
Cerebral palsy	37
Poliomyelitis	10
Spina bifida	8
Heart disease	9
congenital and rheumatic	
Muscular dystrophy	7
Others including:	29
haemophilia, congenital limb	
deformity, Perthe's disease, etc.	

General considerations

Before treating handicapped children it is important to obtain a recent medical assessment. Such information will define the abnormality, the medical treatment including drugs which the child is receiving, and should detail risks that dental treatment might involve. Closely allied with this information are the possible health hazards of a general anaesthetic given, either in the dental surgery or within a hospital.

Generally speaking there are no appreciable differences in caries rates of either subnormal or physically handicapped as compared with normal children, but gingival disease is more common. It is, however, significant that there is a higher proportion of untreated dental caries in the physically handicapped and educationally subnormal.

Not all handicapped children are difficult to treat and many can muster a useful level of cooperation so that small restorations can be carried out satisfactorily. However it is necessary to recognise the limited discomfort tolerance, especially in subnormal children, and treatment should never be continued in a situation where only severe physical restraint by the nursing staff can make the child submit. These are conditions which would be intolerable even for normal children and the fear experienced by those with both intellectual and emotional impairment, of being unprotected against such a physical assault, is not difficult to imagine. The standard of work which is likely to result from the operator's determination to proceed under such circumstances is an eloquent testimony of the need to carry out these restorations under the controlled advantages of a general anaesthetic.

Almost without exception, the results of their own efforts to keep their mouths clean are poor. In cases of severe subnormality and paraplegia, the child must depend for oral hygiene entirely on the help of nursing staff or parents, and this can present serious physical problems where an overweight teenager requires support and toothbrushing at the same time.

The physically handicapped child is said to be one who, over an appreciable period, is prevented by physical condition from full participation in childhood activities of a social, recreational, educational or vocational nature. The child becomes isolated by his disability, and his normal progress through the stages of domestic and community socialisation is severely restricted. In these circumstances the protective role of the mother is prolonged and often intensified. She bears the burden and the responsibility for bringing the child for treatment and it is essential that she be continuously encouraged and supported in the integral part she has to play in the child's dental health.

Handicapped children should be inspected every four months. This enables the dental surgeon to detect new and recurrent dental disease at an early stage and to prevent risks to health particularly in those suffering from such diseases as cardiac abnormalities and diabetes mellitus. Besides this basic function of oral assessment, these visits are valuable opportunities for discussing dental problems with the parent and also for reinforcing the home oral hygiene techniques.

Physically handicapped. There is a great variety of pathological conditions which limit the performance of normal activities severely. Very commonly those who treat handicapped children will find their patients include some who suffer from muscular dystrophy, congenital limb defects, cerebral palsy and spina bifida.

Dental status. A common finding in handicapped children is that they experience an average caries rate, but their gingival condition is worse. This situation may reflect the child's physical inability to clean the teeth satisfactorily, and that the dental condition is likely to be seriously affected if normal chewing is impossible. Food may have to be fed in liquidised form which lacks any detersive action, and poor oral clearance activity allows it to remain on the teeth for prolonged periods.

Dental considerations

The child's dental health will depend upon the amount of home or community care that he receives from parent or nurse. Effective oral hygiene is difficult to achieve if help is restricted, inexperienced, or if the children are uncooperative and difficult to manage. A point which should not be overlooked is the help that can be given by brothers or sisters of the handicapped child. They are often surprisingly effective in sharing this domestic responsibility with the parents.

Children with limb defects such as those due to thalidomide will benefit from the use of an electric toothbrush. Whilst it is true that many acquire an effective gripping technique with rudimentary hands, or even with their feet, efficient brush rotation and control is very difficult especially in the absence of the thumb. Provided the child can grip the electric toothbrush cylinder, all the necessary fine movements can be carried out mechanically (Fig. 6.1). When the brush cannot be held, a suitable clamp-stand will offer a firm basis for toothbrushing practice and every effort should be made to allow the child to be as independent as possible. When the child's physical disability makes him completely dependent upon others for his oral hygiene the electric toothbrush allows the nurse to carry out effective brushing and, at the same time, to control unwanted movements or support the head and shoulders during the brushing.

The following features are desirable in an electric toothbrush:

Safety. The toothbrush must be completely detached from any mains electric source during use. It is not sufficient to have an insulated brush mechanism with a mains power cable attached, since

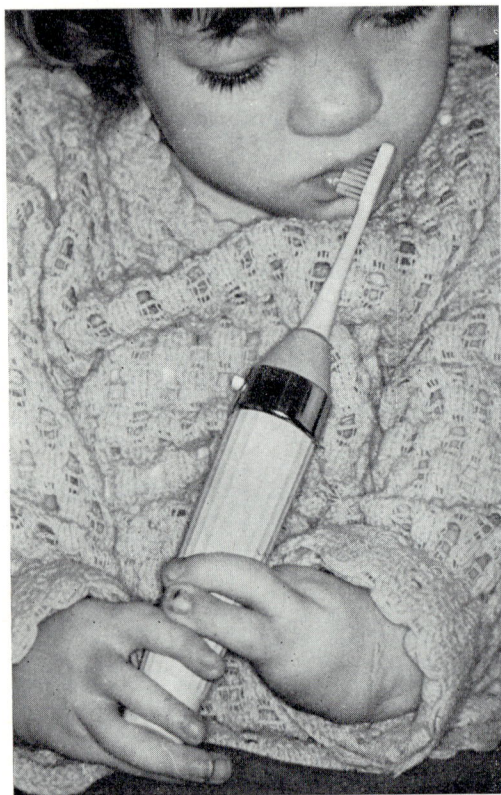

Fig. 6.1. Photograph of child without thumbs, using a two-handed grip on an electric toothbrush cylinder. (Courtesy of General Electric Company U.S.A.)

the latter may become kinked or cut and lead to a highly dangerous situation. Battery operated or rechargeable cell units are safer, but they must be effectively isolated to prevent unpleasant electric shocks and to preserve them from damp corrosion.

Brushing efficiency. Arcuate up and down brush movements are those most difficult to make effectively with a hand brush and most beneficial for cleansing interdental areas. For use in the confined buccal spaces of a child's mouth a small brush head is an advantage, but the tufts must be both firm and pliable.

Design. The casing should be light and streamlined and the switch mechanism sufficiently simple so that it can be switched on without the need for continuous pressure on the switch during use. It is important that the child with hand deformities shall have sufficient length of handle to be able to use both hands on the casing.

When the assessment of the child's physical disability has been made it is essential to demonstrate by use of models and slides the most effective way in which toothbrushing should be done in the particular circumstance. Such simple steps as these, together with dietary factors discussed in Chapter 3, are often neglected, but it should be remembered that these children have special problems of oral hygiene which require individual solutions.

Good cooperation can be expected when the child's physical condition permits. Whilst it is inevitable that many severely handicapped children will require a general anaesthetic for restorative treatment the possibility of using local anaesthesia and appropriate premedication should always be considered. When many extensive restorations are needed, this will be a factor influencing the decision whether to use general anaesthesia. There is a tendency, once the child is known to be a 'restorations under G.A case' to leave small cavities found at inspection until several can be done at the same time. This attitude is unfortunate in that it tends to neglect the importance of prevention of dental disease and also deprives the child of the opportunity of graduating to a treatment acceptance level where small single restorations can be carried out. The value of this to the child's self-esteem is enormous and can provide a much more optimistic basis for future treatment.

Disadvantaged and Emotionally Inadequate Children

These children are of average intelligence but lack the emotional development to endure unpleasant situations. They are amongst the most difficult children to treat and their display of parental dependence and overprotection does little to arouse sympathy in the surgery. In some cases their behaviour may reflect difficult home life, but in others it may be emotional stress associated with such disorders as diabetes or epilepsy. It has to be remembered that all children who are physically ill are much less tolerant of discomfort.

Dental status. The dental condition of these children is highly characteristic and reflects every aspect of neglect. Generalised chronic gingival inflammation and a high caries rate are common features. Interproximal caries in young permanent incisors reflects the real gravity of the situation and snacks taken frequently between meals often include biscuits eaten in bed. The parents emphasise how often their child is asked to clean his teeth at home, but further questioning shows that for one reason or another (and there are many) he never quite makes it. In much the same way the child's history is one of unproductive dental appointments, abandoned treatment plans and changed dentists.

Dental considerations. The basis of treatment for these children is to assume that attitude improvements are often possible if they are initially asked to have only simple dental experiences, e.g. scaling and polishing which carry no discomfort. If urgent restorative treatment on many teeth is necessary this work will have to be carried out under general anaesthesia as described at the end of this chapter. It would be intolerable for such children to sit through an operative experience which would daunt most adults. If this rationale of treatment is observed then the balance is temporarily restored in the patient's favour and the child can then look forward to a series of appointments in which the really important tasks of diet and oral hygiene re-education can begin. Oral prophylaxis is gradually introduced as a basis for future operative work. Relapses are common and are to be expected, but the continual reinforcement of the home-help aspects of dental health is essential at every visit. Praise should be given for even small dental achievements both at home and in the surgery.

Local anaesthetics will solve problems of pain but not of emotional inadequacy, but occasionally in older children it is possible to give anxiolytic drugs such as diazepam intravenously together with the use of a local anaesthetic to improve the cooperation. This group contains children who are, however, the least likely to accept local anaesthesia techniques by themselves as a slight preliminary discomfort to allow freedom from pain later on. Generally speaking, premedication offers many advantages, but in considering suitable drugs the following points should be borne in mind:

(*a*) These children are not inpatients but are attending clinics and they must be protected and supervised all the time they are under the influence of the drug. Furthermore, only responsible individuals must be allowed to supervise the actual drug administration. This should never be left, under any circumstances, to the children themselves, no matter how old they may be.

(*b*) These drugs are dangerous and must be kept locked away when in the home, particularly where there are younger children in the family.

(c) The drugs tend to induce degrees of drowsiness and occasionally other side-effects such as amnesia. The parent should be advised when to expect these reactions, how long they are likely to last and what protection should be given to the child during this period of time.

The Subnormal Child

This group includes children suffering from cerebral palsy, mongolism, phenylketonuria, hypothyroidism, hydrocephalus and microcephalus. They are characterised by a low level of intelligence and limited cooperation and, in some cases, have a characteristic appearance. The defect may be present at birth or develop soon afterwards when other associated physical abnormalities may be discovered. Varying degrees of muscle spasticity or rigidity may be present.

Dental status. Adequate oral hygiene and dental care are often lacking with a result that there may be much untreated caries and periodontal disease. The limited cooperation severely restricts the amount of operative work that can be undertaken for these patients and their only dental experience may have been of general anaesthetics for extractions.

Dental considerations. Advantage should be taken of the fact that in milder degrees of subnormality, a limited degree of cooperation can be expected. In some cases this can be augmented to such a level that oral prophylaxis, simple restorations and even limited endodontic treatment can be carried out.

In the older age-group, severely subnormal children may present difficulties in control and cooperation even when simple toothbrushing is attempted. It is in these cases that the electric toothbrush can offer many advantages to nursing staff or parents when attempting to maintain an adequate state of oral hygiene.

The oral hygienist with her special knowledge of brushing problems and her commitment in the child's oral health programme can do much to encourage and recruit the limited cooperation of these children. Inspections should be frequent, because subnormal children possess only a limited ability to communicate and they may have to endure considerable dental pain until the cause is discovered by accident.

The problem of treating fractured incisors should be related to the degree of subnormality and to the expected cooperation. In some cases it is possible to carry out endodontic treatment in the chair where this involves simple removal of a necrotic pulp. In more painful endodontic situations a general anaesthetic will be necessary, but these teeth should not be extracted unless the root canal situation is complicated by prolonged infection or anatomical abnormalities. Even though these children have impaired intellectual abilities, the slightly subnormal are often embarrassed by the loss of front teeth and are very happy to wear and look after a small denture.

Children with Cardiac Disease

The two main groups of heart disease in childhood are rheumatic and congenital. The importance of rheumatic fever lies in the risk that a bacteraemia may at some time during the illness give rise to a carditis which will result in chronic rheumatic heart disease, usually with mitral stenosis. Congenital heart disease includes aberrations of the major vessels, septal and other defects, all of which confer the risk of bacterial endocarditis if the heart is exposed to a bacteraemia. General anaesthesia is a serious hazard to patients with cardiac disease.

Dental status. The state of oral hygiene is generally poor and the high caries rate frequently results in the need for dental extractions. Carious exposures of permanent incisor pulps are not uncommon and constitute a difficult problem of prognosis. The long association with hospital treatment often makes these patients uncooperative.

Dental considerations. Prior consultation is essential before carrying out any form of dental treatment, and a history of cardiac murmers should be regarded with suspicion and confirmation sought. Children who have a history of heart disease or defect should never be treated in a routine manner, no matter how urgent their dental treatment. Cases requiring general anaesthesia should be hospitalised for specialist assessment and supervision during treatment.

Antibiotic cover is essential when disturbing the soft tissues of patients with cardiac disease, including those with a history of rheumatic fever and should be given in the following two stages:

1. *Initial cover:* benzylpenicillin, by intramuscular injection half an hour before dental operation.

250,000 units (1-5 years.)
500,000 units (6-12 years.)

2. *Continuity of cover:* phenoxymethylpenicillin, by mouth every six hours for 3 days after dental operation.

125 mg (1-5 years.)
250 mg (6-12 years.)

The initial intramuscular injection guarantees a high circulating concentration of the antibiotic which can deal effectively with sensitive organisms released during tissue disturbances such as extractions or pulp removal. Although the peak blood concentration is rapidly reached, the benzylpenicillin is quickly excreted and the protection should therefore be continued with the phenoxymethypenicillin capsules.

Cases will arise where, because of penicillin allergy or the occurrence of resistant strains of organisms, alternative forms of antibiotic cover will be required. Medical advice should be sought in this matter, but it should be remembered that tetracyclines taken by mouth are best avoided since they are only moderately absorbed, are not bacteriocidal and have the added disadvantage of discolouring the teeth. If there is a history of sensitivity to penicillin then the following régime is recommended before extractions or scaling:

1. Cephaloridine 0·5-1·0 mg half an hour before hand.
2. Erythromycin 125-250 mg orally four times daily for 3 days.

Alternatively erythromycin 250-500 mg may be given orally 3 hours before treatment, followed by erythromycin 125-250 mg orally four times daily for 3 days.

Children with Haemorrhagic Diseases including Anaemias and Leukaemias

The condition varies greatly with the medical situation, for example, in haemophilia, bleeding occurs after the slightest injury and may continue in submucous tissue or along muscle planes. If this occurs in the face and neck it may lead to respiratory embarrassment and a significant blood loss. In haemophilia the lack of factor VIII can be temporarily remedied by the addition to the defective blood of cryoprecipitate containing antihaemophilic globulin (A.H.G.). The absence of other factors, such as factor IX in Christmas disease, represents failure at other points of the clotting mechanism. Aplastic anaemia and the leukaemias give rise to serious haematological changes which constitute risks of both haemorrhage and infection.

Dental status. These cases present special dental problems when injury or infection are present and particularly if extractions are required.

Dental considerations. A history of abnormal bleeding and clotting always requires investigation before treatment is undertaken. Treatment is designed to restore teeth at the earliest opportunity, together with a thorough supervision of oral hygiene and diet, since only in this way is it possible to avoid the complications following extractions.

No extractions or oral surgery—no matter how minor—should be attempted unless the patient is hospitalised to receive appropriate therapy beforehand. The hospital treatment of extraction sockets should be based on routine procedures. In haemophilia the basis of a firm clot will depend upon intravenous A.H.G. given as cryo-precipitate, and both extensive suturing and chemical applications to the socket should be avoided, since they damage the tissues, increase the risk of infection, and will not produce clotting in the absence of factor VIII. Once the clotting mechanism has been temporarily restored by the addition of A.H.G. there is usually no need to restrict the number of teeth scheduled for extraction. Pre-operative radiographic root analysis and meticulous surgical technique will greatly reduce trauma and risk of infection. Even local anaesthesia should not be used in the dental surgery if the patient has a clotting defect, since this may be followed by prolonged bleeding into tissues. Pre- and post-operative antibiotics by mouth will help to prevent secondary infection (see previous section on antibiotics dosage).

Children with Diabetes Mellitus

Diabetic children present a hyperglycaemia with impaired glucose metabolism. The situation is controlled by diet and insulin therapy, but these children are intolerant of infection which disturbs their insulin control. They require stabilisation before a general anaesthetic is given and are usually admitted to hospital for this purpose.

Dental status. The periodontal condition is poor, with a high rate of calculus formation and chronic marginal gingivitis. The caries rate also tends to be high, despite dietary restrictions. The tissues have a poor resistance to infection which is frequently of dental origin in young children.

Dental considerations. If surgical treatment in the mouth is being considered it should be preceded by scaling and polishing and carried out under an antibiotic cover such as that given above for children with cardiac defects.

The regulation of diabetes is always critical and control is easily lost, particularly if infection or extensive tissue disturbance occurs. For this reason it is preferable to refer cases requiring multiple extractions into hospital so that they may receive the appropriate stabilisation before and after surgery.

Aims of treatment must be:

(*a*) To prevent and eliminate dental infection by early treatment of carious lesions and gingival conditions.

(*b*) To have continual reference to the medical situation in so far as it complicates, or is complicated by, the patient's dental treatment.

Children with Adrenocortical Insufficiency and other conditions requiring Corticosteroid Therapy

Besides adrenocortical hypofunction, there are a number of conditions for which corticosteroids are given, including asthma, hay fever, haemolytic anaemia, idiopathic thrombocytopaenia, nephrotic syndrome, rheumatic fever and skin conditions. Adrenal insufficiency results in a situation where the patients can no longer react normally to infection or stress and this may produce a state of collapse. Acute infection, injury or emotional shock may precipitate such a crisis. An increase in steroid therapy will be necessary until these episodes are passed.

Dental status. Oral infection, trauma, or stress in anticipation of a general anaesthetic or surgical procedures may seriously disturb the patient's steroid balance.

Dental considerations. Medical consultation is essential when treating these patients and increases in the dosage of steroid therapy may be required preoperatively. In most cases it is preferable to refer them to hospital when surgical treatment under a general anaesthetic is necessary, and antibiotic therapy is essential if there is any risk of soft tissue damage since healing is affected by steroids.

Patients with adrenocortical insufficiency are often fretful, but a sympathetic approach helps to reduce their fears and, providing the procedures are not hurried and are accompanied with explanations, considerable cooperation can be obtained. Early treatment where there is minimal caries should be combined with supportive oral hygiene and diet instructions.

Children with Epilepsy

There are over 60,000 schoolchildren with epilepsy in England and Wales. It is a disease which may present in a variety of ways from grand mal with frequent major seizures to petit mal where there is only momentary loss of consciousness. The presence of abnormal electrical patterns of the brain is implicit in the diagnosis of epilepsy and the fits require control by anticonvulsants, i.e. phenytoin (Epanutin) and phenobarbitone. These drugs may be necessary throughout life but primidone (Mysoline) may be used instead of phenytoin and has advantages of control without causing gingival hyperplasia although it is not suitable for all cases.

Dental status. The caries rate is average and the poor gingival condition is associated with a hyperplastic gingivitis (see Fig. 2.18). Falls during epileptic attacks are frequent, fractured incisors are common, and loss of teeth may lead to drifting and malocclusion in upper labial segments (Fig. 6.2).

Dental considerations. These patients should always be accompanied by an adult and never left unattended in the surgery or waiting-room.

Epileptic Fit

All chairside assistants and clinical attendants should know what to do if a fit occurs:

1. Push aside all moveable equipment including trollies and bracket tables, and summon assistance.
2. Support head and shoulders and ease patient from the chair on to the floor on his back as quickly as possible.
3. Padded tongue spatulas should be wedged between upper and lower buccal teeth. If this is done quickly it will help to prevent injury to tongue and teeth.
4. Other assistants should gently restrain active limb movements and prevent their injury.
5. Patient's jaw is kept supported and head turned slightly to one side to ease control and prevent respiratory embarrassment.
6. These children are distressed following an epileptic attack and need sympathetic understanding and reassurance.

Neither partial dentures nor orthodontic appliances should be considered for these cases unless they have been free from fits for at least eighteen months. In many cases malocclusion, due to crowding, can be alleviated by planned extractions.

Fractured incisors are common and every attempt should be made to preserve these teeth and avoid the difficulties of wearing a prosthetic replacement. Sensitive dentine should be covered with a stainless steel protection cap and exposed pulps treated routinely as described in Chapter 5. Following this initial treatment either three-quarter crowns or basket crowns should be constructed for the fractured tooth.

Oral hygiene is poor and this is to a large extent associated with the phenytoin hyperplasia of the gingivae. Local control can be effected by vigorous brushing, preferably using an electric tooth-brush. If, however, the gingival tissue is greatly enlarged then

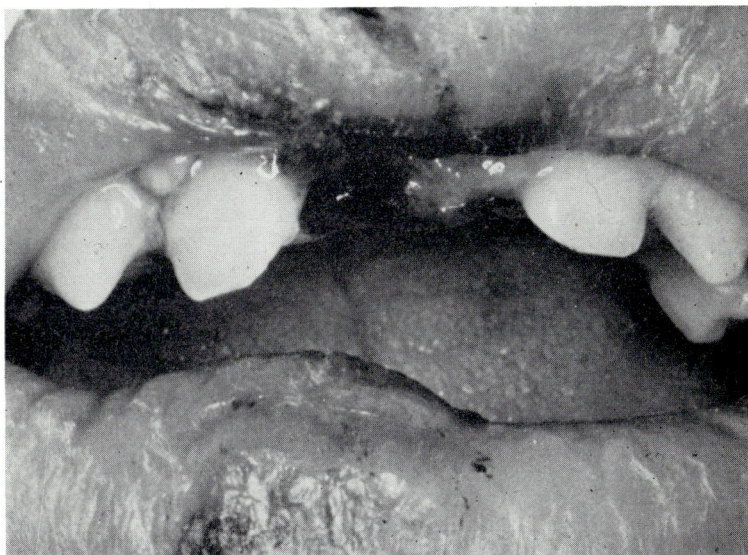

Fig. 6.2. Photograph recording the earlier traumatic loss of /1 and recent luxation of 1/ with associated lip injuries. Such cases illustrate the prosthetic problem where an upper denture cannot be worn to prevent the drift of 2/2, unless the epilepsy is controlled.

gingivoplasty may be necessary and may have to be repeated from time to time as the condition tends to recur. This surgical treatment is carried out under a general anaesthetic and an acrylic or silver splint used to secure zinc oxide-based gingival packs during the first week of healing.

Restorations under General Anaesthesia

General anaesthesia in relation to dentistry is undergoing considerable changes in both scope and techniques, but the decision to use a particular method must always be an individual one which takes account of the patient's need and safety. The use of intravenous diazepam as an anxiolytic drug has had considerable success, but the methods described in this section are intended for patients where techniques such as those using premedication or intravenous sedation together with local anaesthesia have either failed or are unsuitable, and they have therefore particular reference to the treatment of many handicapped children already described.

General considerations

The aim of this method of treatment is to carry out all dental procedures whilst the patient is anaesthetised, and these will sometimes include endodontics and extractions. In severely handicapped children it may be necessary to carry out all treatment in this manner, so that two sessions of approximately forty-five minutes each may be required to produce a state of dental fitness.

Dental debris presents a high-risk factor for the unconscious patient in the horizontal position and it is necessary to protect the child's airway by intubation using a cuffed tube. Careful attention should also be given to protecting the child's eyes and this is best provided by applying a layer of padded gauze as soon as the child is anaesthetised.

The use of high-speed cutters and diamonds which can be regarded as essential in this type of work, means that a large volume of water will collect in the packs unless the spray control is kept at a miser level. A powerful and efficient sucker together with a reserve are essential and, if a wide nozzle is used, it can be strategically placed to collect dental spray and debris directly from the cutting area.

Dental considerations

Preliminary. A good dental assessment is necessary before making arrangements for carrying out the operative work under a general anaesthetic. This is of great value, since the operator will have to decide the following:

1. The way in which the dental treatment and anaesthetic are likely to affect the patient's health is especially important for those suffering from such diseases as diabetes or cardiac defects. Discussions with the anaesthetist and physician may indicate that a prolonged anaesthesia is contraindicated and that only urgent dental conditions may be attended to. Treatment priorities will then have to be adjusted to fit these circumstances.

2. The dental surgeon has to decide how cooperative his patient is likely to be and whether it will be possible to obtain preoperative radiographs of, for example, the periapical condition of fractured or severely carious permanent incisors. If they cannot be obtained he must decide how far he can usefully proceed, using clinical evidence alone, at the time of treatment. The preparation of teeth for jacket crowns presupposes that they can be cemented at a later routine appointment.

3. Precise notes should be made of the teeth requiring treatment, and the type of restorations most suitable. Such restorations may not, of course, take their final form at this stage as in those cases requiring Class III amalgams in lower incisors, but these may be replaced at a future time if there is improvement of cooperation and oral hygiene. Generally speaking this restorative treatment is confined to the permanent dentition and very carious primary teeth are extracted.

4. As the operator completes his assessment his requirements for instruments and materials will become evident together with his needs in terms of operating and ancillary staff. His work programme should be related rigidly to the patient's capacity for treatment and subsequently to his recovery and after-care.

Finally, the patient and all those who are to be concerned in the treatment should receive adequate preparatory instructions and information.

Operative. Nasal intubation is preferable to an oral tube since the latter can seriously limit the available working space once the tube is in position, the oro-pharynx is packed off with continuous ribbon gauze and a sponge pack. Any loose primary teeth are removed before the prop is placed in its working position. It is an advantage to slightly dampen the dry packs with saline before insertion, as this avoids soreness of the oro-pharynx afterwards. Once the tube and packs are in position, the airway is protected by three continuous but independent systems. If unpredictable vomiting should occur then these will have to be withdrawn at speed whilst the unconscious patient is being rapidly tilted from a horizontal to a head-downwards and sideways position. In this event the operator will find it an advantage to devise a simple plan when packing the oro-pharynx, so that the free end of the ribbon gauze and the securing line of the sponge are extended out of the mouth and easily located in a pre-arranged position.

The restorative work is usually carried out in segments beginning with the most posterior cavities in the lower arch. Generally it is preferable to cut all the preparations in that segment before the filling materials are inserted, but this plan may have to be abandoned if unexpected endodontic situations such as pulpotomy or pulp-capping become necessary. If extractions are unavoidable, they should be left until the treatment in the corresponding upper segment is completed, otherwise the operative field will become obscured with blood.

The sponge pack should be examined frequently and replaced if it becomes saturated. If an oral tube is being used it may require re-positioning once treatment on one side of the mouth is completed and it may be an advantage to repack the whole of the oro-pharynx at this stage to avoid kinking the tube.

Care will be needed in positioning rubber props over any teeth which have just been restored and it is worth bearing in mind that these segments should be re-examined for possible damage before the anaesthetic is lightened.

Endodontic complications, following trauma or caries may occur in immature teeth and in those with complete apices. The value of preoperative assessment radiographs has been mentioned and they can indicate the best line of treatment in the situation. It may be necessary for instance to carry out an apical root resection for long-standing periapical lesions and not infrequently adjacent incisors may also be involved so that preparations can be made to include both teeth in the surgical treatment. A recent exposure of a vital immature pulp should be treated by partial pulp amputation (pulpotomy) as described in Chapter 5. If, however, there is no bleeding from the pulp chamber the contents will be seen to be necrotic and should be extirpated. Excessive pulpal bleeding indicates hyperaemia which may have passed into an irreversible stage so that the pulp's recovery is doubtful. When this situation arises, even in the immature incisor, it is preferable to remove as much of the pulp tissue as possible, and allow time for fluid drainage whilst attending to other incisors. The endodontic therapy should then be completed, and the canal filled with absorbable paste and sealed with zinc phosphate cement and amalgam.

Emotionally disturbed and subnormal children may not tolerate even such simple procedures as impressions for partial dentures. Where necessary these can be carried out as part of the programme to be completed under a general anaesthetic. The poor cooperation of the child may prevent the preparation of special trays before hand, but facsimilies made from thermoplastic base-plate material are easily preformed on old plaster models of appropriate size. Close adaptation can be carried out by heating the tray in a bowl of hot water, and after testing for temperature shaping directly on the oral tissues. Whenever possible the tray should extend posteriorly to include the 1st permanent molars, so that Adams' cribs may be included on the denture to improve its retention.

The impression is recorded in alginate, which is fixed to the tray surface coated with adhesive. Before the impression is recorded the props and gags must be removed and the patient sufficiently relaxed so that the jaws can be gently separated to admit the loaded tray. As the tray is seated in position care must be taken to control and remove the excess impression material. Since an occlusal registration is not possible at this stage the final incisor relationship must be assessed preoperatively and adjusted at the wax try-in stage. Finally, the tooth shade should be recorded.

7 Incisors: Abnormalities and Aesthetics

The appearance of the incisors is of great importance to the patient who may attend principally because of their unsatisfactory position, shape or colour. Fortunately these abnormal situations can be substanially improved by treatment, providing the patient is willing to cooperate. Even when only small changes can be achieved, these often result in a great increase in the child's confidence and feeling of social acceptance. Occasionally, the coronal defect may be so disfiguring that the only satisfactory solution is the provision of a jacket crown.

Treatment of Hypoplastic Teeth

Preventive measures

The close relationship between the apices of BA/AB, and the underlying permanent crowns means that the latter are liable to show hypoplastic defects following trauma or apical infection of the primary teeth. The two points that should be stressed when chronic infection occurs in primary incisors, are that endodontic therapy should be avoided, and these infected teeth should be extracted.

Operative treatment

Small single hypoplastic defects may be filled with little difficulty although aesthetic restorations on the flat exposed enamel surfaces of 21/12, require considerable skill in matching resins or silicates. When the defect lies in a background of mottled or blemished enamel then a matching plastic restoration becomes almost impossible. Much depends on the severity of the mottling, but it may be so disfiguring that the only satisfactory solution is the provision of a jacket crown.

Generalised enamel hypoplasia due to systemic disturbances requires special consideration because of the following features:

(a) Even though $\dfrac{21/12}{21/12}$ may be severely affected there is much aesthetic improvement when only 21/12 are crowned.

(*b*) Where the horizontal line of defects weakens the crown its fracture is likely to occur unless a jacket crown is constructed.

(*c*) The teeth may be immature, but secondary dentine will usually permit jacket-crown preparation with minimal pulp disturbance.

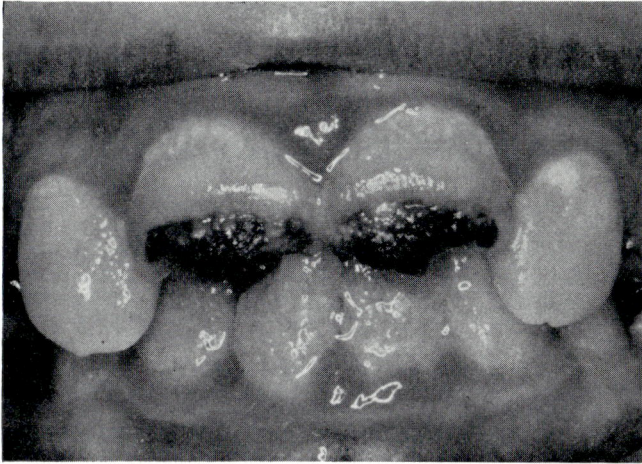

Fig. 7.1*a*. (*a*) Hypoplastic defects 1/1 crowns.

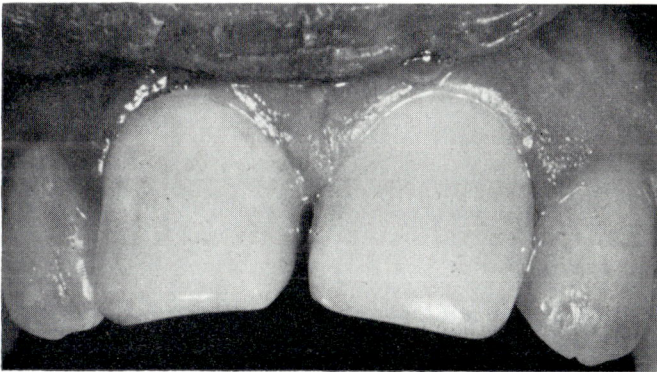

Fig. 7.1*b*. (*b*) Acrylic jacket crown restorations on 1/1.

Enamel hypoplasia may allow rapid wear of incisors and buccal teeth, and should be treated with jacket crowns (Figs. 7.1*a*, *b*) and shell crowns respectively to prevent further attrition. Fortunately it is more usual to find that these types of restorations are necessary only for the 1st permanent molars and 21/12, but one should bear it in mind that extensions to the jacket-crown preparations will be required as the child grows into late teenage and early adulthood, to take into account the elongation of the clinical crown.

Treatment of Discoloured Teeth

Intrinsic discoloration

In dentinogenesis imperfecta, slender, brittle roots may be present so that preoperative radiographs are essential in order that the root form of each individual tooth may be anticipated. Treatment of these cases concerns itself with two features:

(*a*) Prevention of excessive wear in primary and permanent teeth.
(*b*) Aesthetics of the permanent dentition.

It is necessary to anticipate treatment in an immediate and a long-term phase so that steel crowns or cast silver caps may be used initially to prevent excessive wear and unpleasant thermal stimuli of the primary teeth.

When the permanent incisors erupt the construction of shoulder-less jacket crowns will restore their aesthetics in cases of generalised defective enamel. These should be constructed for 21/12 as soon as there is any evidence of excessive wear, but in hypoplastic incisors where the defects are localised these may be replaced by individual restorations, and a conventional jacket crown made in the late teenage period, if the appearance demands it.

Preconstructed proprietary stainless steel crowns should be used for hypoplastic 21/12 and left in place until jacket crowns can be constructed at sixteen years of age. In the case of hypocalcified permanent molars and premolars the construction of shell crowns should be delayed until eruption is complete but as an intermediate stage, stainless steel crowns or cast silver caps may be constructed to prevent wear.

Discoloration following pulp injury

Primary incisors. Great care should be exercised when deciding to retain upper primary incisors which have darkened following injury. Even though these teeth may be symptomless, periapical inflammation may result in a hypoplastic patch on the labial aspect of the underlying permanent incisor. There is evidence to suggest that the rapid fading of initial discoloration of primary incisors indicates that the tooth, despite its trauma, has retained its vitality, so that internal resorption of the blood pigment can occur.

In any case radiographs should be taken within four to five weeks, since these may show evidence of periapical bone rarefaction indicating inflammatory changes, and under these circumstances the primary tooth should be extracted. No attempt should be made to carry out endodontic therapy on these incisors for fear of injury to the underlying permanent incisors already mentioned.

Permanent incisors. Where the dentine is deeply stained following the breakdown of pulp tissues two possible lines of treatment are available and these consist of either bleaching or crowning the tooth.

Bleaching is only successful in a limited number of cases. Long-standing stains are much more difficult to treat. Before bleaching is undertaken all endodontic treatment should have been completed and a well-sealed root filling placed in position.

1. Isolate the tooth with rubber dam.
2. Remove all carious and stained dentine and old fillings.
3. Using a No. 8 rose-head bur remove the root filling to the level of the cervix.
4. Thoroughly dry the internal aspect of the crown using 70 per cent alcohol together with warm air before sealing in the perhydrol (30 per cent hydrogen peroxide in water), on a cotton pledget which is left for ten minutes. Renew the solution, seal in and repeat after forty-eight hours. This method may be used in conjunction with an ultra-violet beam to accelerate the bleaching action. However, unless there is a significant improvement following the second application, then further bleaching is unlikely to produce satisfactory results and an alternative of a post crown should be considered.

CROWNING. Whether a jacket crown or post crown is constructed depends on the quality of the remaining tooth tissue. If the crown is fractured or extensively weakened by the endodontic preparation, then a post crown is preferable.

Tetracycline staining

Prevention. If possible the use of systemic tetracyclines in children should be avoided, especially in the first seven years of life. All tetracyclines will stain the developing teeth and it is essential to give alternative antibiotics such as erythromycin where there is a penicillin allergy or resistant infections. Except where enamel hypoplasia is present, the teeth are of normal form although stained. The treat-

ment is therefore concerned entirely with aesthetics and in severely
stained teeth the only effective means of disguising their appearance
is by means of a jacket crown. However, the situation requires careful analysis before hand to determine just how much the stain disturbs the patient. If possible, crowning should be postponed until
the late teenage period, and in the first instance confined to the upper
incisors.

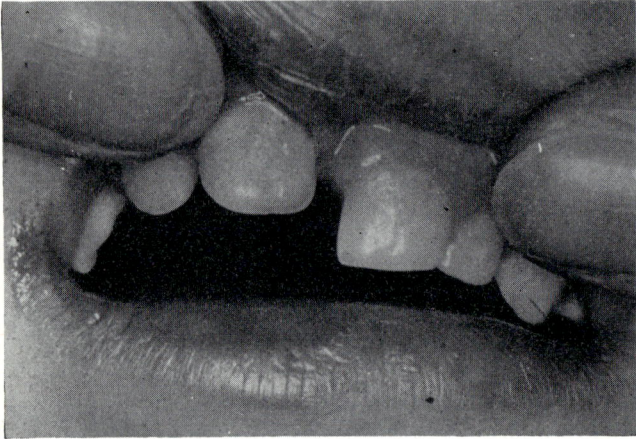

Fig. 7.2. Irregularity of primary incisors due to digit sucking.

Caries discoloration

Local loss in translucency especially in proximal and occlusal
areas may indicate an underlying carious lesion. Sometimes internal
discoloration may give the crown a bluish-brown colour, but exposed
carious dentine becomes a dark brown.

Treatment consists of caries removal, but if this leaves an extensively weakened tooth, a jacket or post crown may be necessary to
restore the appearance satisfactorily.

Brown and black discoloration

Certain stains are not associated with neglected oral hygiene and
many disappear after a thorough scaling and polishing. However,
they can be prevented from returning if the enamel is cleaned with a
fine sandpaper disc and painted with 2 per cent solution of sodium

fluoride. Two such courses are usually necessary to obtain a lasting result.

Orthodontic Conditions

Malocclusion in the primary dentition

Variations in the occlusion of the primary dentition, although less frequent, reflect the same range of abnormalities which can be found in the permanent teeth.

Crowding and spacing. A midline diastema may develop when A/A, erupt, but this usually closes when CB/BC appear. In some occlusions the spaces persist either in the incisor area or throughout the entire arch. Sometimes crowding of the anterior teeth may occur in such a way that B/B are lingually placed with A/A protruding.

Irregularities in the incisor area may be aggravated by sucking habits (Fig. 7.2), including the use of 'comforters'. These habits tend to produce retroclination of lower incisors and associated irregularities in the lower labial segment. At the same time, the BA/AB may be proclined. In the primary dentition an anterior open bite is usually due to soft tissue influence and not to skeletal abnormality.

Absence of primary teeth is rare, although it may be in evidence to a marked extent in ectodermal dysplasia where there is usually considerable spacing within the arches (Fig. 7.3a, b).

Incisal relationship in the deciduous dentition. A Class I incisor relationship is seen in the majority of children. The extremes of Class II division 1 are seen in the Pierre Robin syndrome with its associated defect in the cranial base angulation, although in the majority of cases this tends to be self-correcting by the age of four years.

Milder forms of Class II division 1 incisal relationships are common but are aggravated by digit and lip sucking. Although Class II division 2 incisal relations are not so frequently seen they usually show less retroclination of labial segments than does the same situation in the permanent dentition, and are without the periodontal complications due to gingival trauma at a later age.

Class III incisor relationships may be seen in cases where centric occlusion is achieved and also where there is a forward displacement of the mandible during closure. Following the premature loss of primary molars there may be an initial contact on $\frac{C/C}{C/C}$ causing forward mandibular displacement in order to chew and this may result in a Class III incisor relationship.

TREATMENT. Where initial contacts are interfering with centric

G

occlusion (see Chapter 2) grinding or extraction of teeth may be indicated to allow a free range of jaw movements.

Although there are possibilities for correcting a crossbite in the

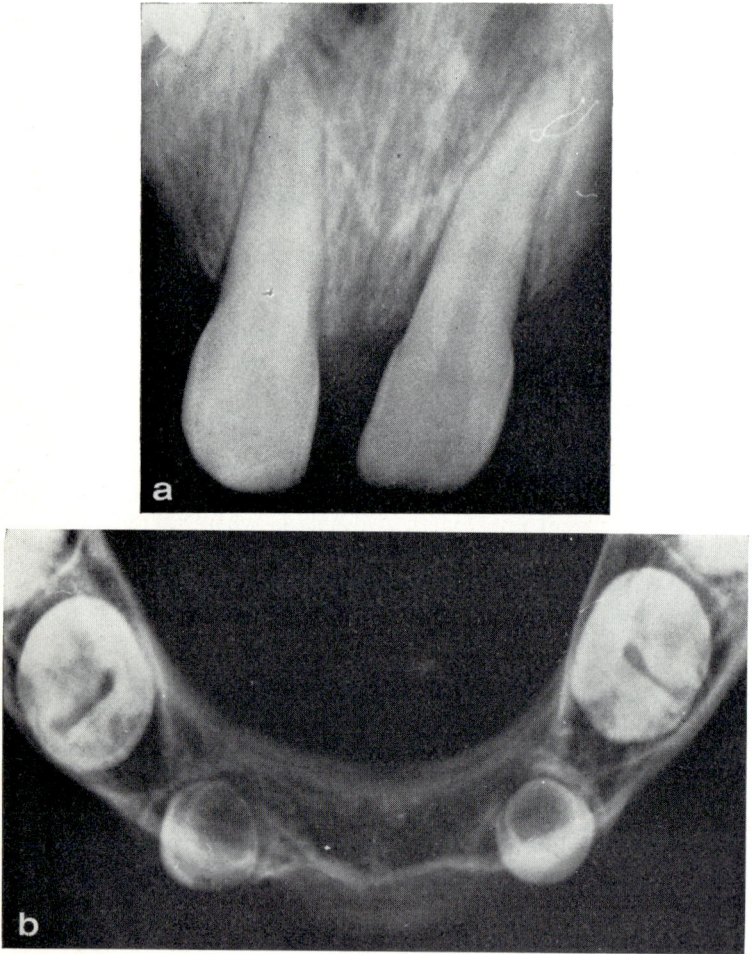

Fig. 7.3*a* and *b*. Radiographs showing partial anodontia of (*a*) upper and (*b*) lower incisor areas of a child with ectodermal dysplasia.

buccal segments of the deciduous dentition it is not always possible to maintain this improvement in the successional teeth. Correction of Class II division 1 incisal relationship in the primary dentition is of doubtful value, since it will not eliminate the need to treat in the permanent dentition at a later date. Malocclusion in the primary dentition should be accepted except in cases where eccentric occlusion can be corrected by occlusal grinding or extractions.

Malocclusion in the mixed dentition

Anterior root-crowding phase. This well-known developmental appearance which, unfortunately, used to be described as 'the

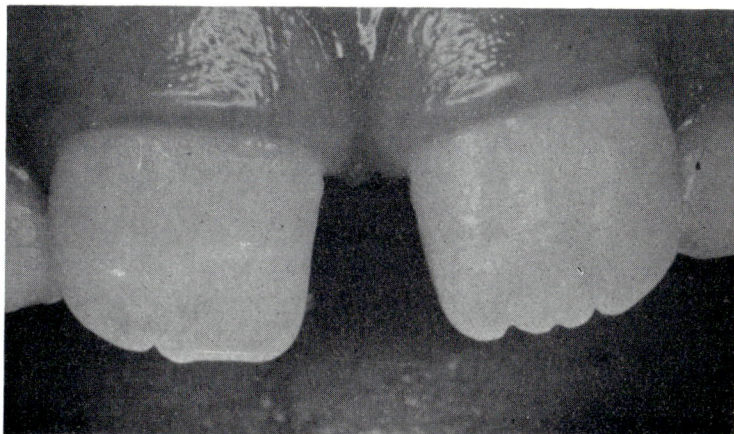

FIG. 7.4. Crown spacing showing characteristic separation of 1/1 due to root crowding of these teeth by the erupting 32/23.

ugly duckling' phase, refers to a state of root-crowding and crown-spacing in the permanent incisors, where 21/12 are present but 3/3 have not yet erupted. When the 3/3 are moving occlusally they cause the roots of 21/12 to be compressed leaving the crowns free to spread laterally. This may be especially noticeable between 1/1 (Fig. 7.4). The labial midline frenum is prominent and it has been suggested that frenectomy is necessary to allow 1/1 to approximate. However, with the average tooth to bone-tissue ratio or where the mouth is crowded, eruption of 3/3 enables closure of the 21/12 spaces and regression of the frenum without surgical intervention. In fact this condition may be accepted as a phase of normal development and it is reassurance of the anxious parent that is called for, rather than appliance therapy.

Central diastema. The central diastema (Fig. 7.4) may be part of the anterior root-crowding phase of development already mentioned, or on the other hand there may be a bodily spacing of the 1/1 due to an intervening maxillary bone suture, separated by a fibrous tract which may be an extension of the labial frenum. Evidence of the separated suture can be seen radiographically. It may be a symptom of generalised spacing, a condition where the teeth are small in relation to the size of the dental base (Fig. 7.5) and

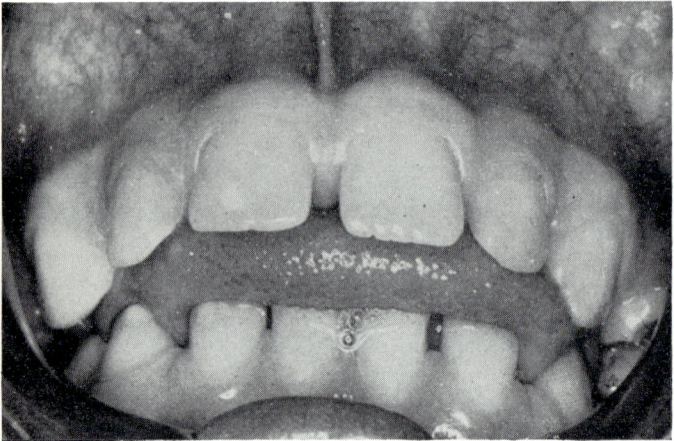

FIG. 7.5 Generalised spacing in upper and lower dental arches where there is a discrepancy between tooth size and arch size.

includes cases of partial anodontia and diminutive 2/2. It may be due to supernumerary teeth mechanically preventing approximation of 1/1 (Fig. 7.6.) Thumb sucking may also bring about a separation and proclination of 1/1.

TREATMENT. Supernumerary teeth should be removed and 1/1 approximated where necessary using fixed appliances to achieve root movement. Frenectomy should be carried out following tooth movement so that the contraction of fibrous scar tissue maintains the approximation of 1/1.

Partial anodontia. The 2/2 or $\dfrac{5/5}{5/5}$ are the teeth most commonly absent. Third molars may fail to develop in a number of cases, but this may not be apparent radiographically until the child is nine years old. The absence of 2/2 may allow a diastema between 1/1, but this depends on the tooth to bone-tissue ratio. In most cases when the 3/3 erupt the resulting pressure causes approximation of 1/1. If, however, space persists, the use of fixed appliances is indicated to localise the space, followed by provision of a partial upper denture to retain the alignment of the teeth and improve the appearance. In certain Class II division 1 types of malocclusion, absence of 2/2 may permit overjet reduction without the need for extraction and produce an acceptable result.

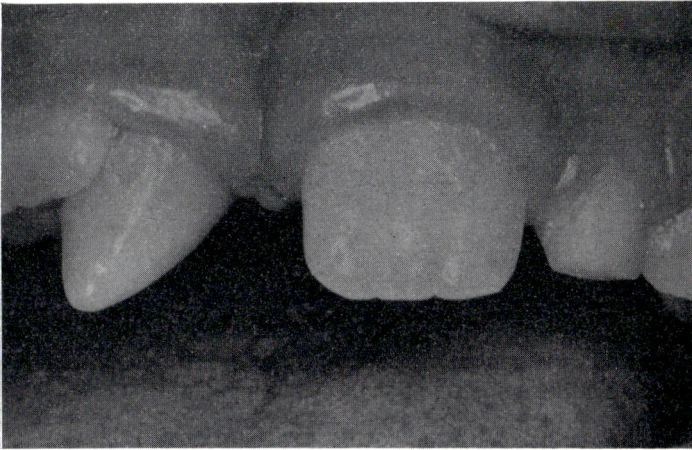

Fig. 7.6. A supernumary tooth separating 1/1

In the lower arch with absence of 52/25, the occlusion may be improved by the approximation of 31/13 and provision of a partial denture in the premolar area.

Treatment of Teeth of Abnormal Form

Dens invaginatus

All abnormal incisors should be radiographed before attempting treatment.

Palatal pits should be restored with amalgam, the cavity preparation being carried out only in the superficial part of the pit. No attempt should be made to cut a cavity deeply within the crown invagination as the abnormal internal anatomy may lead to the exposure of unexpected superficial pulp tissue. The more extensive the invagination the greater the dilatation of the crown to the extent that its proportions may interfere with the occlusion. Because of the internal abnormalities of extensively invaginated teeth, crown reduction or endodontic treatment is impossible so that extraction followed by a partial denture may give the only satisfactory solution.

Dilacerated incisors

Unless the deflection of the root is in the apical one-third and accessible for surgery, extraction is usually the only effective treatment and should be followed by provision of a partial denture or closure of space by means of a fixed orthodontic appliance (Fig. 7.7).

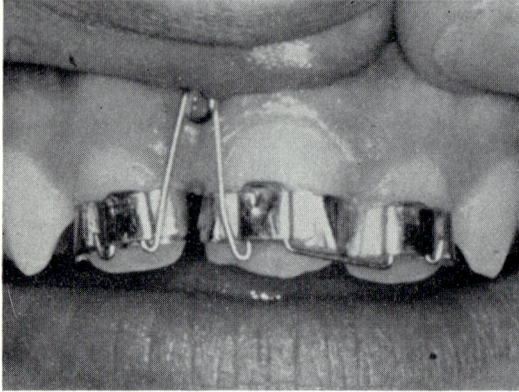

Fig. 7.7. Use of a fixed orthodontic appliance to move 2/ into 1/ space.

Diminutive incisors

Jacket crowns will satisfactorily restore the majority of diminutive incisors providing the root is sufficiently robust, but the spacing between adjacent incisors will require closure by orthodontic means before the width of the jacket crown can be accurately assessed. Care must be given to the cervical finish of the crown so that its contour is compatible with healthy gingival tissue.

Treatment of geminated incisors

The patient often seeks an improvement in appearance and attempts may be made to groove the labial and incisal edges so as to simulate separate adjacent incisors. The grooving must be shallow and attempts to divide the wide crown axially should be avoided, since even with good radiographs, pulp damage and exposures often occur.

In the majority of cases the width of the geminated incisor complex produces crowding in the labial segment. The same situation arises where an incisor carries additional cusps (Fig. 7.8). If this crowding is severe, its relief may be produced by extraction of adjacent poorly positioned teeth or teeth in the buccal segments. The decision to extract other sound teeth for this purpose should be delayed until the useful, functional, and aesthetic life, of the geminated tooth is certain.

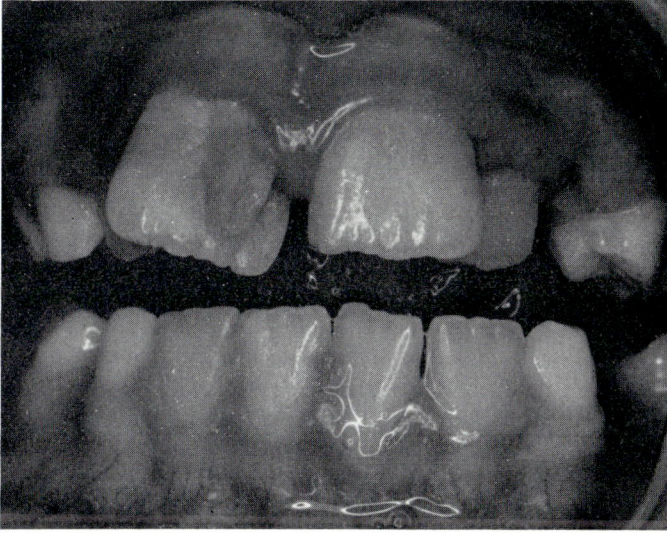

FIG. 7.8. An incisor crown with additional cusps.

Non-eruption of anterior teeth

If either or both upper central incisors remain unerupted when 2/2 are breaking the mucosal surface, early radiographic investigation is called for. Failure of both 1/1 to erupt often indicates the presence of supernumerary teeth (Fig. 7.9), but failure of one or other central incisor suggests that this may be due either to a supernumerary tooth or a malformed root.

Clinically the situation is investigated by palpating the area to attempt to locate the presence of supernumerary teeth. Subsequently periapical films are taken to show the root form followed by a vertex occlusal view to locate the supernumerary tooth on the buccal or palatal aspect of the arch. A postero-anterior skull view is also of

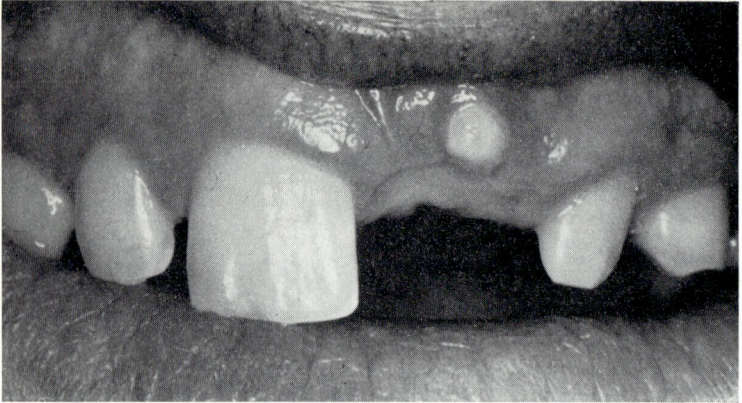

FIG. 7.9. A supernumerary tooth preventing the eruption of a
central incisor.

value in this respect in order to show the vertical position of the
supernumerary tooth in relation to the occlusal plane.

Occasionally, impaction of the upper canines, lateral and central
incisors may be the cause of non-eruption of the incisor teeth (Fig.
7.10*a, b*).

TREATMENT. Surgical removal of supernumerary teeth is indicated, and depending on the information gained from radiographic
examination, a buccal or a palatal approach should be adopted.
The supernumerary tooth should be removed with minimal disturbance of adjacent teeth and, at the same time, bone removal
should be confined to the palatal aspect. The removal of buccal
bone is likely to lead to a permanent irregularity of the gingival
margin of the permanent incisors. After this surgical procedure time
should be allowed for the natural eruption of the central incisor. If,
however, after nine months, there is no sign of this occurring, the
incisor should be re-exposed, fibrous tissue removed from the palatal
aspect and the area packed to encourage the tooth to erupt. Alternatively, a soft wire noose may be placed around the neck of the
tooth so that traction may be applied. Odontomes require surgical
removal, and the provision of a partial denture or closure of space
using orthodontic appliances when a tooth of the permanent series
is involved.

Cleft lip and palate cases

Patients born with a cleft of lip and palate usually show a disturbance of the dentition (Fig. 7.11). This is more likely where the

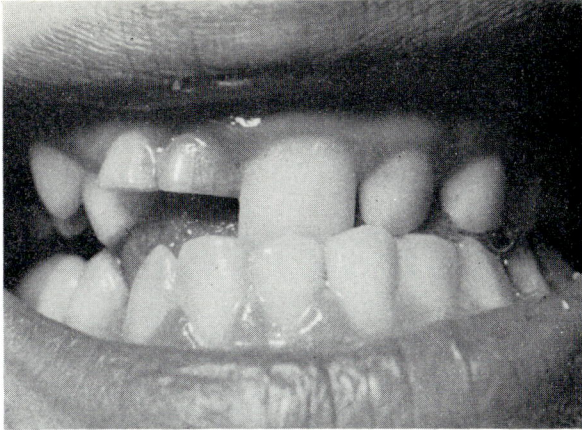

a

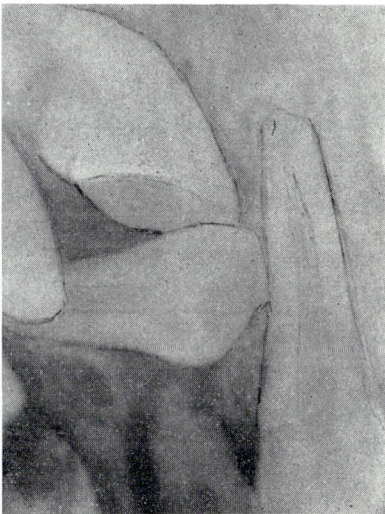

b

Fig. 7.10a and b. Impaction of 3/ and 1/

(a) Clinical photograph of retained BA/.

(b) Underlying impaction of 1/ with 3/ preventing eruption of 21/.

cleft involves the alveolus, but where it affects the lip only there may be a disturbance in alveolar development not clinically apparent in the early years.

It is usually found that where the cleft involves the alveolus the upper lateral incisor is absent in the deciduous series and the upper deciduous canine in erupting, does not develop to the correct occlusal level. This is true in unilateral and bilateral clefts. In cases where

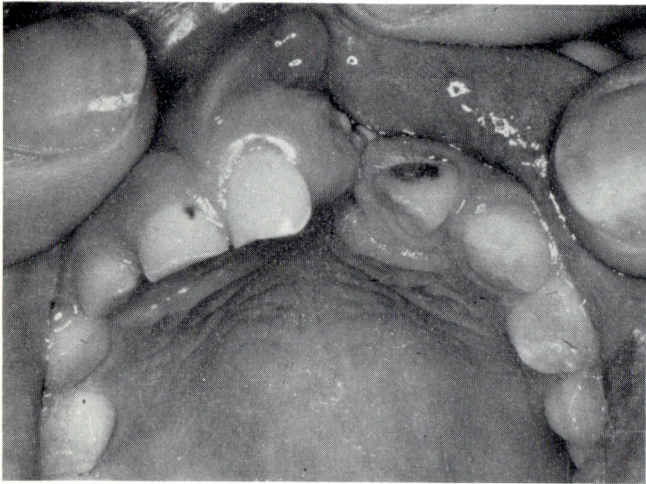

Fig. 7.11. Disturbance of the occlusion due to cleft of aveolus and palate.

there is either a complete or incomplete cleft of the lip, supernumerary or supplemental upper deciduous lateral incisors may appear.

In the permanent dentition the cleft may result in a missing upper lateral incisor tooth combined with rotation of the upper central incisor on the affected side. There is a lack of development of the upper canine on the affected side so that this tooth does not reach the occlusal level and has a palatal inclination. Where there has been a cleft of the alveolus it is known that there is a failure in continuity of mesodermal tissue and unless this can be successfully replaced by a bone graft it is not possible to move teeth into the line of the cleft.

TREATMENT. It is the aim of orthodontic treatment in these cases to align the remaining teeth and replace the missing lateral incisor with a partial denture. Fixed appliances are invariably required to correct the rotated teeth and at the same time a palatal collapse of teeth in the lesser segment can be corrected.

In cases where there is a cleft of the lip only and a missing lateral incisor with an intact alveolus showing only a small fibrous defect, the remaining teeth in the arch may be moved along and adjusted in order to close the gap providing there is initial crowding. This avoids the need for a partial denture.

Other irregularities common to any patient with a malocclusion may also be found in cleft cases and should be treated on the principles of general orthodontic practice.

Malocclusion in the permanent dentition

Relief of crowding. Essentially, crowding of teeth is due to a disproportion between the amount of tooth substance and the amount of bone which is available to accommodate them. It is commonly noticed that certain teeth are excluded from the arch more frequently than others, for example, upper canines and lower 2nd premolars. This is because these teeth usually have to erupt between standing teeth in the arch. The impaction of 3rd molars is also a symptom of crowding. They often become impacted because they are the last teeth to erupt, and therefore the available space has already been taken up by other teeth in the arch. Crowding will be relieved by extraction of permanent teeth. Before these are extracted, however, it is important that a full radiographic investigation of the mouth is made in order to locate all unerupted teeth and ensure that they are of good quality and in a favourable position to erupt. It is particularly important that this is observed not only in the case of the upper canine but also for the lower 2nd premolar because of the way in which this tooth is occasionally found to be hypoplastic (Fig. 7.12) or grossly lingually displaced. The other factor to consider in lower premolar extractions is the degree of distortion of the crown in a mesiodistal direction (Fig. 7.13), as these teeth may require a greater arch length than usual. Radiographic examination will aid in assessing the degree of caries affecting teeth in the area and the presence of suspected periapical disease or abnormal root-form which will seriously influence the decision as to which teeth should be extracted.

In considering relief of crowding it is advisable to discuss individual teeth, commencing with the incisors.

Central incisors. It is rare to advise extraction of upper central incisors for relief of crowding, as their loss adversely affects the patient's appearance. However, in the lower arch, loss of a lower central incisor may be indicated where the remaining incisors are root-crowded and the single incisor is outstanding, the latter often suffering loss of gingival attachment.

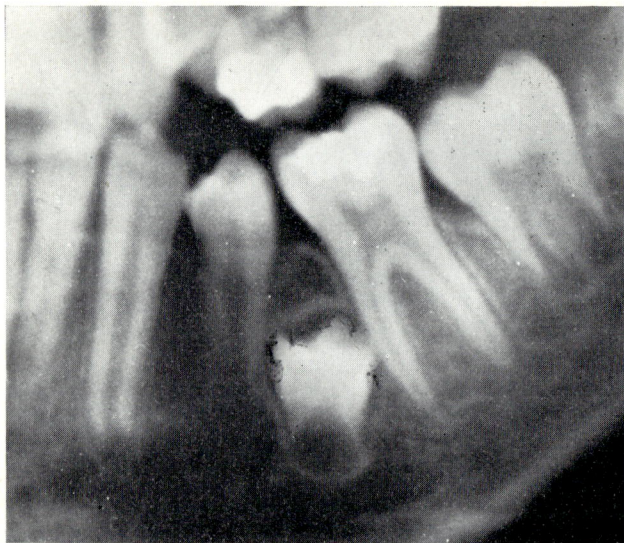

FIG. 7.12. Hypoplastic crown of unerupted $\overline{/5}$.

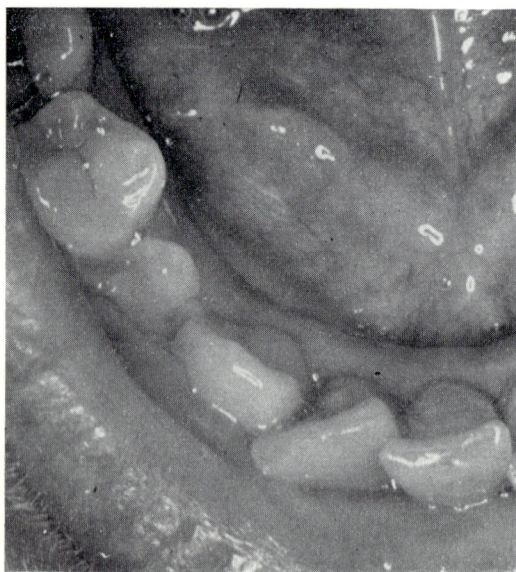

FIG. 7.13. $\overline{5/}$ with increased mesiodistal dimension.

Where the loss of a lower incisor is to be considered, the general rule to apply is that the most upright tooth should be removed to allow the adjacent tilted teeth to straighten into better axial positions. It is the authors' opinion that extraction of a lower incisor tooth before eruption of 2nd molars can lead to a very unsatisfactory result (Fig. 7.14) because the eruption of 2nd molars, and sometimes

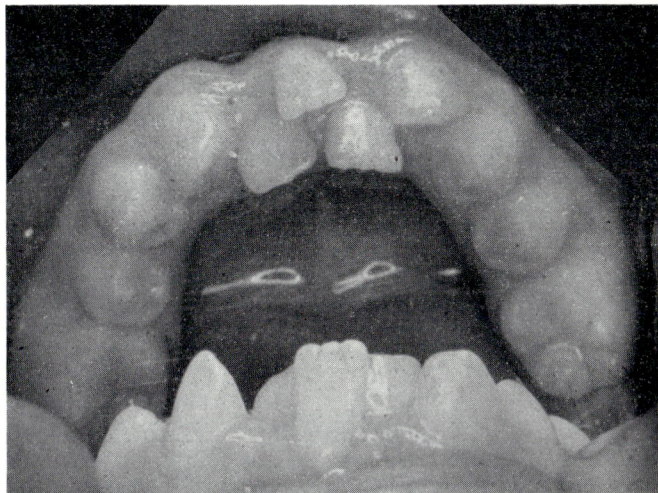

Fig. 7.14. Unsatisfactory result after premature extraction of a lower incisor in a severely crowded lower arch (viewed in mirror).

premolar teeth, introduces further crowding. In cases where there is an irregularity of the lower incisors during this early stage of development, no matter how straightforward it may appear to remove one of these teeth, there is no doubt that the most satisfactory method of treatment is extraction of appropriate premolars followed by appliance therapy to align the incisor teeth.

Lateral incisors. Extraction of lateral incisors may be indicated in cases of crowding in the upper arch where the lateral incisor may be of good form but completely palatal to the arch with the canine adjacent to the central incisor. Loss of the upper lateral incisor may also be indicated when it is hypoplastic or diminutive and where the opposite lateral incisor is absent. Although a more symmetrical appearance is achieved in this way, it should be remembered that the arrangement of 31/13 may not produce a good occlusion because of the large canine cingula. Occasionally where there has been transposition of a lateral incisor and canine, loss of the upper lateral incisor may be indicated. In cases where the canine root is mesially placed its accommodation in the arch may be easier if the upper lateral incisor is removed.

Canines. Loss of the upper canine must be considered when the upper lateral incisor and 1st premolar are in contact and the canine is excluded either buccally or palatally placed. Extraction of the canine must also be considered when it is grossly misplaced (Fig. 7.15)

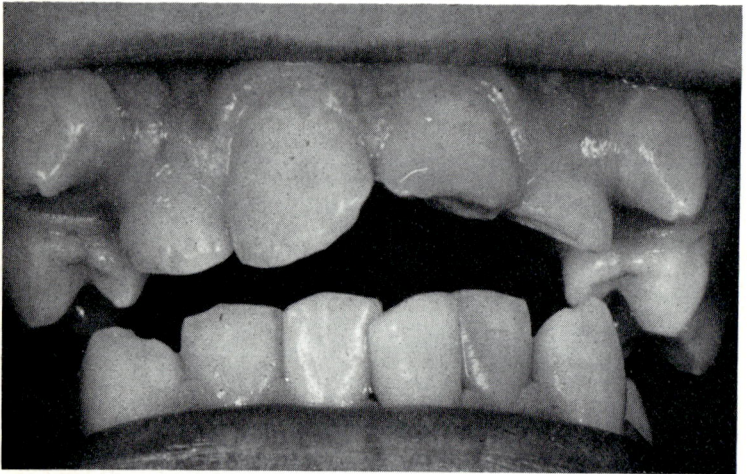

FIG. 7.15. Severe crowding where 3/3 are excluded 21/12 imbricated, and 5/5 are palatally placed or impacted.

from the arch with insufficient space available for its accommodation by orthodontic tooth movement or transplantation. It is important in all cases when considering loss of upper canines to ensure that the upper 1st premolar is not rotated and only shows its buccal aspect. Otherwise a poor cosmetic result will be achieved. Loss of the lower canine is indicated when it is grossly misplaced, for instance horizontally and buccal to the roots of the lower incisors. In cases of transposition it may also be necessary to consider loss of canine teeth.

Premolars. Where canines are slightly excluded from the arch, where there is mild imbrication of the upper anterior teeth in Class I incisor relationship, extraction of 1st premolars will allow accommodation of the remaining teeth by tooth drift without resort to appliance therapy. In the lower arch where 2nd premolars are impacted, loss of 1st premolars will allow these teeth to erupt and improve the occlusion. If the impacted 2nd premolar is removed, an ugly space will subsequently exist between the 1st premolar and the 1st molar, leading to a deterioration in the periodontal condition. Loss of 2nd premolars is rarely indicated, but there are instances where these teeth are lingually or palatally excluded from the arch and here it is the tooth of choice for extraction to relieve crowding.

1st Molars. The relief of crowding by the extraction of 1st lower molars but without resort to appliances must be undertaken by the dental age of nine years. This allows the 2nd molars to erupt into a satisfactory position. If the 1st molars are lost at a later stage, the

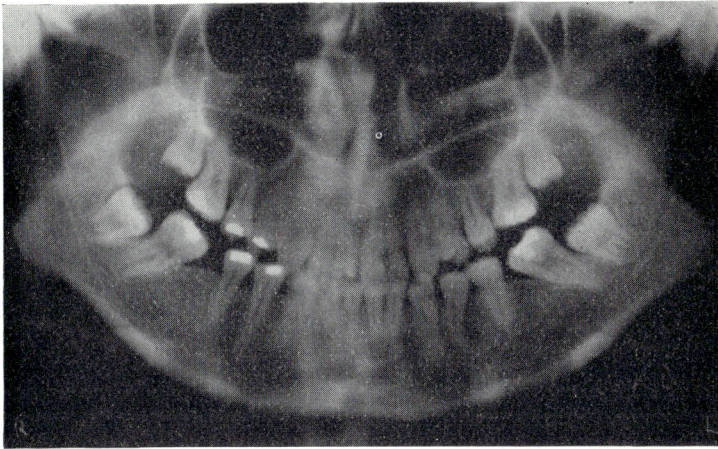

Fig. 7.16. Radiograph showing unfavourable position of $\overline{7/7}$ which have tipped forwards following the extraction of $\overline{6/6}$

2nd molars are likely to tilt forward and produce a very unsatis-factory relationship with the 2nd premolars (Fig. 7.16). Before con-sidering extraction of the 1st permanent molar it is important to ascertain whether the 2nd premolar is distally inclined. Should this be the case it may erupt distally and prevent forward movement of the 2nd molar, eventually leaving a space between the lower pre-molar teeth (Fig. 7.17).

Loss of upper 1st molars in Class I incisor relationship frequently relieves crowding successfully. Extractions should be carried out prior to eruption of the 2nd molars and during the eruptive phase of the premolar teeth. Extraction of upper 1st molars encourages alignment of upper canines, but any relief of imbrication of upper anterior teeth is unlikely, without the use of appliances. The erup-tion of the upper 2nd molars provides adequate space closure and

minimal disturbance of the occlusion, although these teeth tend to
rotate forward to some extent about their palatal root.

2nd molars. Loss of lower 2nd molars in order to relieve impaction of lower 2nd premolars is indicated when there is one-third
of a unit of space discrepancy in the lower arch and when the
lower 3rd molar is favourable for eruption; that is, lies with its

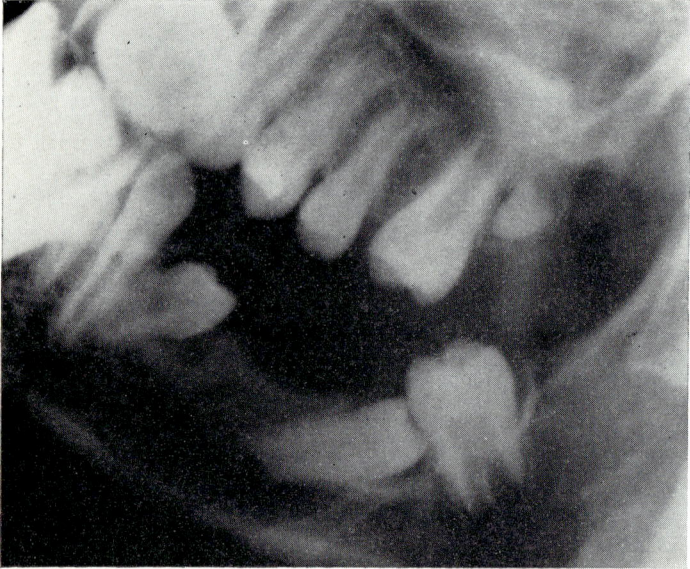

FIG. 7.17. Distally inclined 2nd premolar preventing the forward
movement of the 2nd molar and leaving a space between premolars.

occlusal plane at an angle of 50° or less to the occlusal plane (Fig.
7.18).

Loss of the upper 2nd molars in order to relieve crowding is
rarely indicated, unless appliance therapy is being considered to
retract the buccal segments or for retraction of 1st molars to
accommodate premolar teeth. This will be considered in a later
section.

Traumatic injury to proclined incisors

Proclined upper incisors, associated in Class II division 1 malocclusion with poor lip posture, are liable to injury in childhood (for
predisposing factors see Chapter 5). One should, therefore, consider whether an early treatment of the overjet might reduce the

risk of traumatic injury to the upper incisors. In these cases it would be possible to start treatment at eight and a half to nine years by extraction of C/C and retraction of 21/12. As this would result in loss of 3/3 space, D/D and later 4/4 would require extraction to provide the necessary room for the permanent canines.

Although this scheme of treatment can be very successful, it has two disadvantages. The first of these is that orthodontic treatment has to be extended over a five-year period and the potential advan-

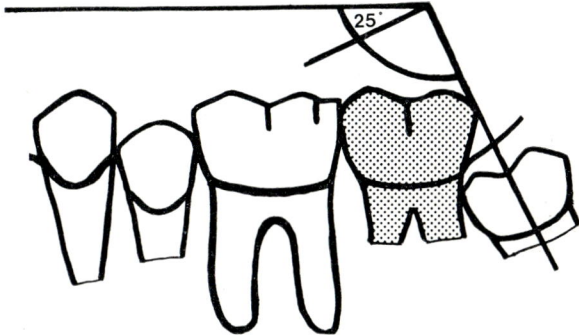

Fig. 7.18. Diagram showing a situation which is favourable for the extraction of the 2nd molar to relieve the impaction of lower 2nd premolar.

tages may be lost because the patient and parent lose interest and abandon the appliance therapy.

The second disadvantage lies in the potential damage to tooth surfaces when appliances are worn for long periods. Enamel decalcification frequently occurs and if the oral hygiene becomes defective there is an increase in dental caries and periodontal disease. Since there is a greater risk of injury to these teeth during sporting activities it is reasonable to construct gum shields as a temporary protection on these occasions. The prognosis of teeth with traumatic injuries in orthodontic cases is considered in Chapter 8.

Class I Incisor Relationship

Treatment is requested in this group for rotated teeth, those having poor axial inclinations and those excluded from the arch by crowding. Occasionally when teeth are spaced, localisation of the space is required, distal to the canine. An upper central diastema with root spacing may be present and will require a fixed appliance

ABNORMALITIES AND AESTHETICS

200

for correction if it persists after 3/3 have erupted. Initially, however, it is necessary to investigate for the presence of supernumerary teeth in the area.

Factors influencing treatment

The dental base may be Class I or mild II, or mild III. The inclination of incisors will be within the range of normal relative to the maxillary and mandibular planes, with an average maxillary mandibular plane angle. Since the labial segments are in soft tissue balance this factor need not be considered as the labial segment position will remain unchanged during treatment. The major consideration in this group is relief of crowding.

The overbite may be incomplete or complete. In order to align the upper incisors, however, it may be necessary during the early part of the treatment to produce an incomplete overbite and this is accomplished by incorporating a flat anterior bite plane (Fig. 7.19*a*, *b*) in the upper removable appliance. Unless this incomplete overbite is initially achieved the anterior teeth cannot be satisfactorily retracted into a position of stabilty relative to the lips.

Treatment of crowded lower arch

Where the lower incisors are imbricated and $\overline{3/3}$ overlap $\overline{2/2}$, loss of $\overline{4/4}$ is indicated, to allow distal drift or retraction of $\overline{3/3}$ and alignment of $\overline{21/12}$. The residual space may be closed by Class II traction. If $\overline{6/6}$ have a poor prognosis these teeth should be extracted when $\overline{7/7}$ have erupted, so the $\overline{54/45}$ and $\overline{3/3}$ may be retracted to allow $\overline{21/12}$ alignment under soft tissue influence. Should the space for $\overline{5/5}$ be inadequate by approximately 2 mm it is advisable to extract $\overline{7/7}$ to allow distal drift of $\overline{6/6}$ and accommodation of $\overline{5/5}$. This also encourages accommodation of $\overline{8/8}$.

Treatment of upper arch

Mild crowding. The indications are a slight imbrication in 3/3 area in which these teeth erupt just buccally to the arch, or alternatively the 5/5 may erupt in a palatal position.

TREATMENT. The 5/5 should be extracted and an upper removable

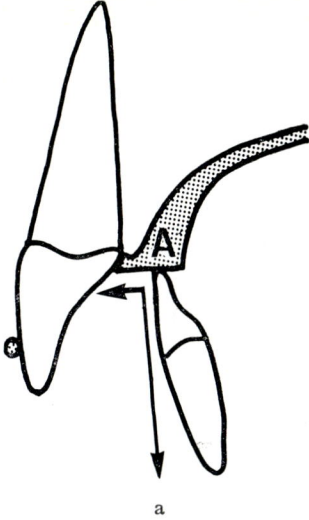

a

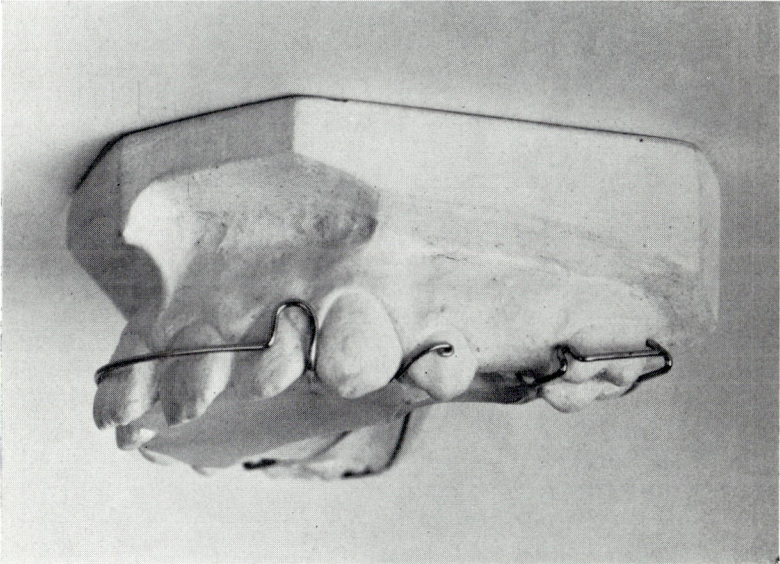

b

FIG. 7.19. (*a*) Diagram illustrating a flat anterior bite plane (A).
An upper removable appliance designed to produce an incomplete overbite as a preliminary to aligning the upper labial segment.
(*b*) Photograph showing an anterior bite plane on an upper removable appliance.

appliance constructed to retract 4/4 and align 3/3 if they are excluded (Fig. 7.20).

An alternative but more lengthy treatment is to extract 7/7 and retract the upper buccal segments distally (Fig. 7.21 *a, b*). Such a plan will not only allow for the alignment of 5/5 or 3/3, but will also provide the opportunity for treating mild crowding of 21/12. If these anterior teeth are rotated however, a fixed appliance will be needed so that the teeth can be realigned in an over-rotated position,

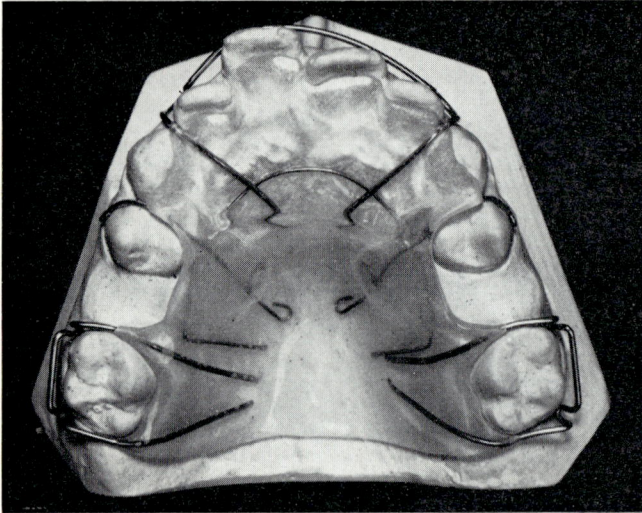

Fig. 7.20. A upper removable appliance to retract 4/4.

(Fig. 7.22*a, b*) in order to compensate for the inevitable relapse which occurs in these cases. A stable result can usually be obtained if the tooth is retained by an appliance for a period of nine months in its corrected position.

Average crowding. Common indications are buccally placed 3/3 with irregularities of 21/12.

TREATMENT. The extraction of 4/4 followed by retraction of 3/3 should be followed by alignment of 21/12 with a removable appliance (Fig. 7.23). Fixed appliances may be needed to treat rotated teeth or correct their axial inclinations.

Severe crowding. In these cases the 3/3 are frequently excluded from the arch and 21/12 may be crowded and irregular. The 5/5 may be palatally placed or impacted (Fig. 7.24).

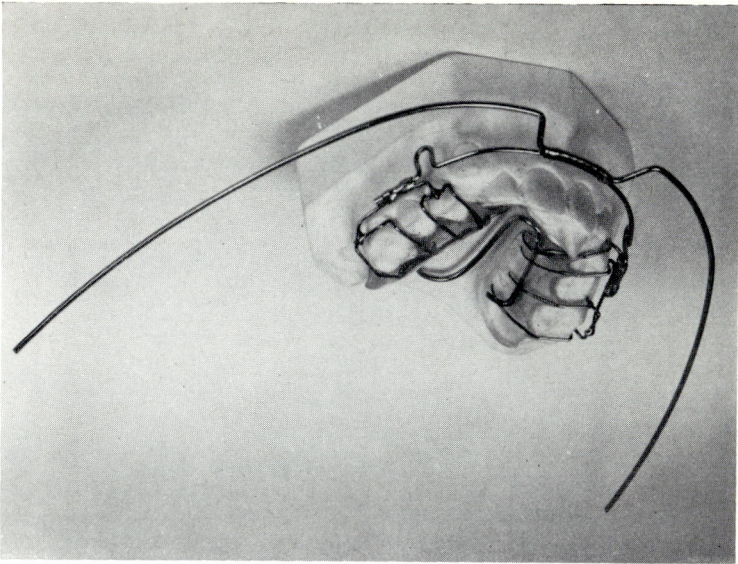

a

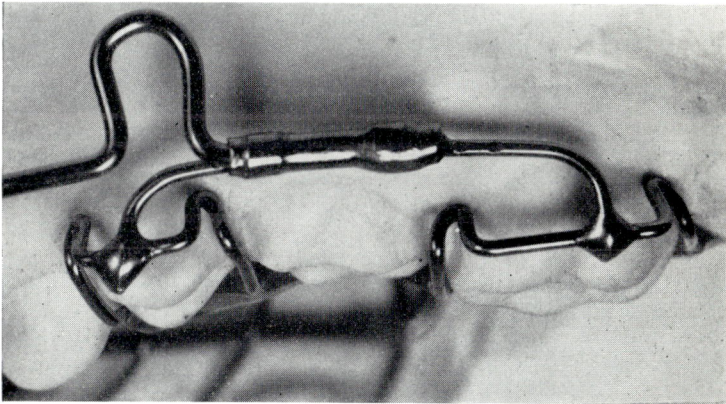

b

Fig. 7.21. (a) Photograph illustrating an upper removable appliance designed to retract the buccal segments by means of extraoral traction applied cervically.
(b) Insert shows details of the attachment of the extraoral bow to the appliance.

TREATMENT. Providing evidence has been obtained that 8/8 are present, the 7/7 should be extracted and the 6/6 retracted to accommodate 5/5 (Fig. 7.25). It is usually advisable to support the appliance with extraoral anchorage (Fig. 7.26). After this has been accomplished the 4/4 are extracted, followed by retraction of 3/3 to allow alignment of 21/12 (see Fig. 7.23).

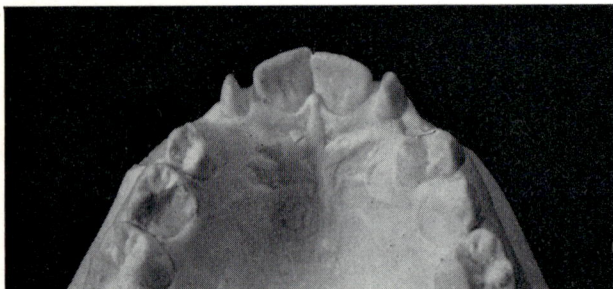

a

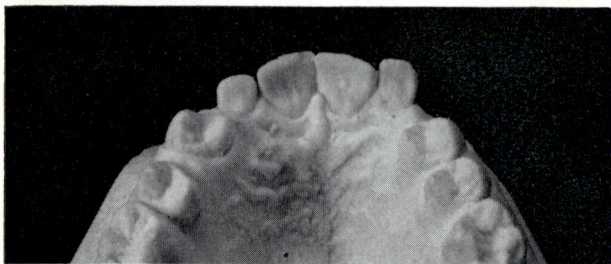

b

FIG. 7.22a Treatment of rotated 2/2 Before appliance therapy.
b. Treatment of rotated 2/2 after appliance therapy (over-rotation).

Bimaxillary proclination

Ideally, this requires treatment by extraction of $\dfrac{4/4}{4/4}$ to allow up-righting of teeth in upper and lower labial segments, with fixed appliances, and should only be undertaken by those who have considerable orthodontic experience.

Spacing of teeth

General spacing can be aesthetically acceptable when there is a distance of 0·5 mm between individual teeth. However, if it is

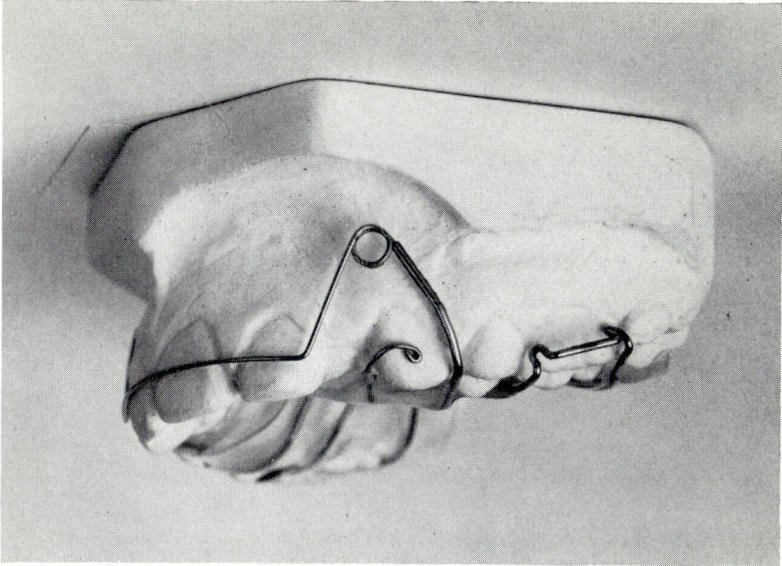

FIG. 7.23. Upper removable appliance to align 21/12.

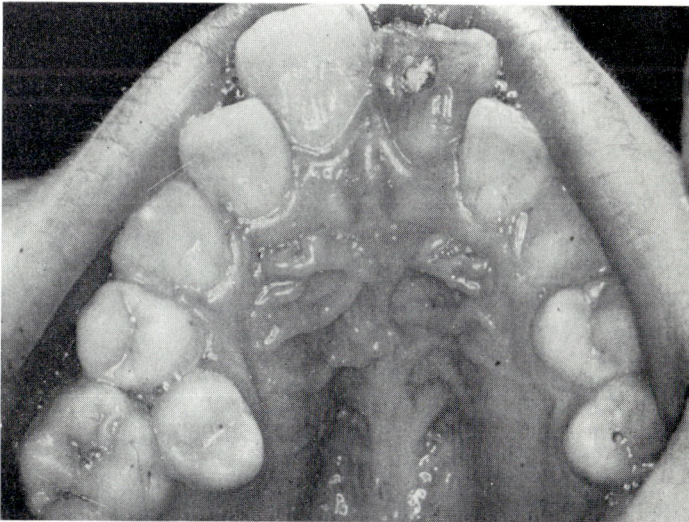

FIG. 7.24. Severe upper arch crowding.

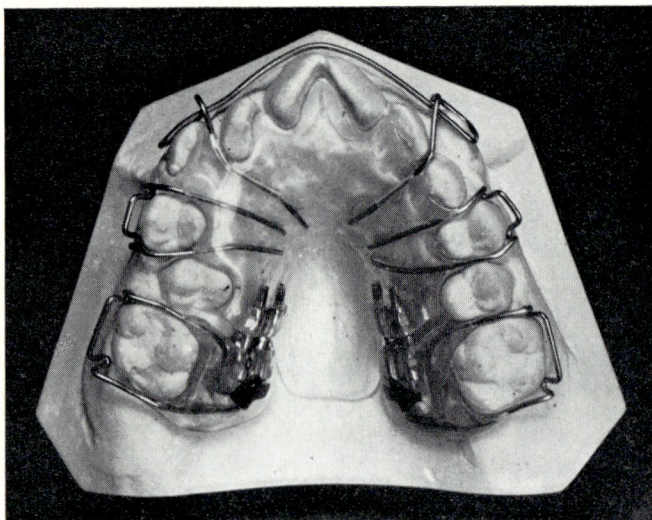

FIG. 7.25. Upper removable appliance with screws to retract 6/6 after extraction of 7/7.

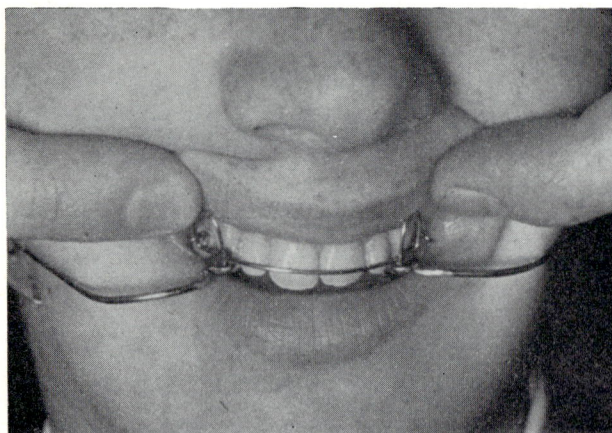

FIG. 7.26. Extraoral anchorage for an upper removable appliance.

greater than this, some space closure may be desired. In such cases fixed appliances will be needed so that tooth movement can be achieved whilst retaining the correct axial inclination. A partial denture and later a bridge in the buccal segments is required to maintain the new relationship of the anterior teeth.

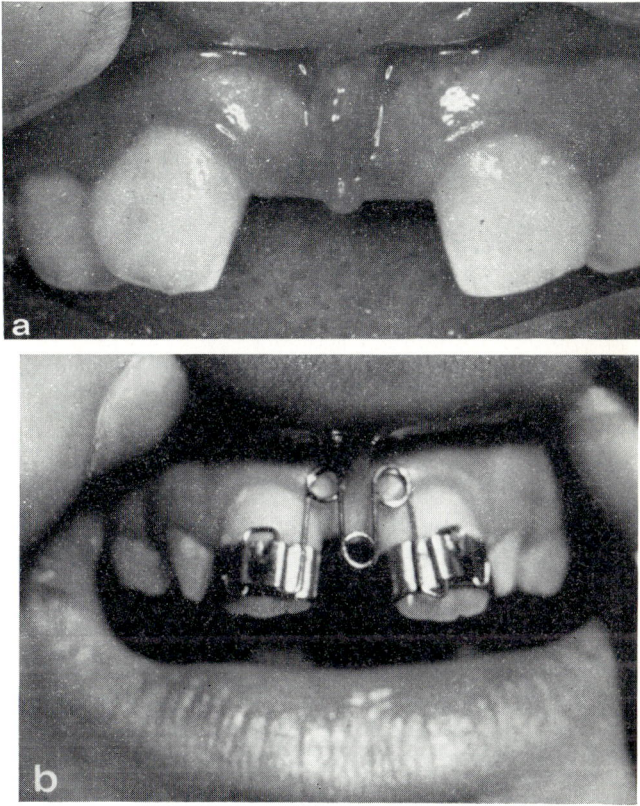

Fig. 7.27. *a.* Central diastema 1/1.
b. Loop and tube fixed appliance to approximate 1/1.

Spacing may be confined to a central diastema (Fig. 7.27*a*) and in these cases treatment should be directed towards approximating 1/1 by bodily movement and not merely tilting the crowns. Fixed appliances such as the loop and tube design (Fig. 7.27*b*) will be required to accomplish this result, but if root-torque or rotation of other teeth is needed then a full multiband technique should be employed.

An anterior open bite may occur in patients with a Class I dental base relationship where the incisor relationship would otherwise have been Class I or a mild Class III. Where the soft tissue pattern is the causal factor, then treatment should include correction of the anterior open bite. However, where it is due to failure in skeletal development no attempt should be made to close it by extraction of teeth in the buccal segments.

Class II Division 1 Incisor Relationship

Treatment in this group aims at correcting the prominence of the front teeth and is the commonest condition for which treatment is requested by the patient. The upper anterior teeth may be spaced, crowded and rotated and the lower arch may also be crowded.

Factors influencing treatment

The dental base relationship may be Class I where the increased overjet is accounted for by proclination of the upper labial segment and/or retroclination of the lower labial segment. Where the dental base relationship is Class II, the degree of overjet is determined by the discrepancies of the dental bases, combined with the inclination of the upper and lower labial segments. If an aesthetically acceptable result is to be achieved in cases where an increased overjet is associated with an upper labial segment of average inclination or even where it is retroclined relative to the maxillary base, then treatment should be carried out with fixed appliances. In these cases the need to 'depress' the lower labial segment is determined by the degree of overbite.

The soft tissue pattern may contribute to the incisor relationship and it should be accepted that habitual tongue thrusts will disappear during treatment. However, whole-time retention must be instituted until the thrust is discontinued so that stability is assured. Relapse occurs when the tongue thrust habit cannot be broken, but this situation rarely occurs. Expressive behaviour of the lower lip may retrocline the lower incisors and in these cases the position of the lower labial segment should be accepted since only partial reduction of the overjet is likely to be achieved by treatment.

Lower arch treatment

Where the lower incisors are imbricated and $\overline{3/3}$ overlap $\overline{2/2}$, the $\overline{4/4}$ should be extracted to allow distal drift or retraction of $\overline{3/3}$

and alignment of $\overline{21/12}$. The residual space may be closed by Class II intermaxillary traction. If, however, $\overline{6/6}$ are of poor quality they should be extracted when $\overline{7/7}$ have erupted, so that $\overline{54/45}$ and $\overline{3/3}$ can be retracted to allow $\overline{21/12}$ alignment under the influences of the soft tissues. If the $\overline{5/5}$ spaces are inadequate by approximately a quarter unit, it is advisable to extract $\overline{7/7}$ to allow distal drift of $\overline{6/6}$ and subsequent accommodation of $\overline{5/5}$. The extraction of the $\overline{7/7}$ also provides space for the $\overline{8/8}$. Where lower fixed appliances are being used in combination with upper removable or fixed appliances the reduction of the overbite is achieved by 'depression' of $\overline{21/12}$ which carry bands that can be used for this purpose. Intramaxillary traction is necessary in these cases so that proclination of $\overline{21/12}$ is avoided. Rarely this movement needs to be combined with bodily lingual movement of the lower incisors, but this requires expert appliance handling with the use of Edgewise arches or the Begg technique suitably modified to suit the lower arch.

Upper arch treatment

Mild crowding. A slight increase in the overjet is sometimes accompanied by rotation of the anterior teeth and there may be an associated buccal segment crowding with $\underline{3/3}$ overlapping the labial segment, or exclusion of $5/5$.

TREATMENT. The $\underline{4/4}$ are extracted and this is followed by retraction of $\underline{3/3}$. At the same time an incomplete overbite is produced using a flat anterior bite plane incorporated into the base-plate of the upper appliance. The $\underline{21/12}$ are retracted whilst the overbite reduction is maintained.

If the $\underline{21/12}$ are rotated or if their inclination to the dental base demands it, a fixed appliance will be required to over-rotate and correct the axial inclination of the teeth. Alternatively, bodily movement may be undertaken to give $\underline{21/12}$ an acceptable appearance (Fig. 7.28), but either the Begg or Edgewise system of fixed appliance therapy will be necessary to achieve such a result (Fig. 7.29).

Average crowding. The indications of average crowding are that either $\underline{3/3}$ or $\underline{5/5}$ have been excluded from the arch by half a unit (approximately 3 mm) and that there is an increase in overjet. One full unit's space will have to be provided in each upper buccal segment to remedy this situation.

TREATMENT. The 4/4 should be extracted and the 3/3 retracted with an upper removable appliance incorporating a flat anterior bite plane to provide an incomplete overbite. Alternatively, a fixed appliance may be used. It is essential in these cases that the buccal

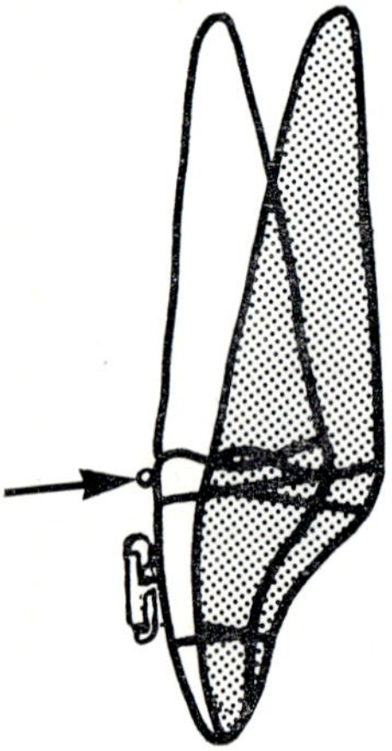

FIG. 7.28. Diagram of bodily movement of an incisor.

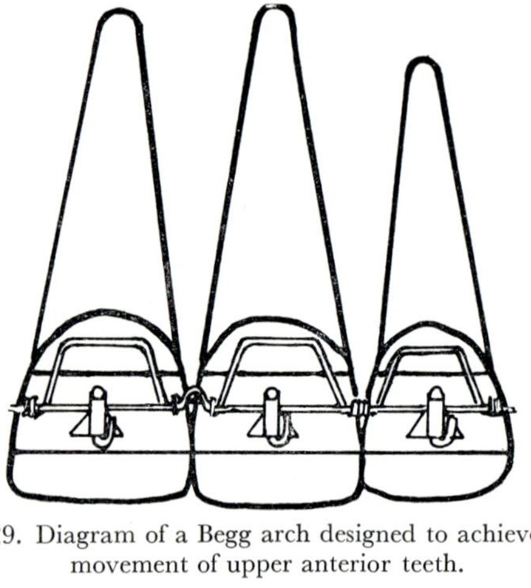

FIG. 7.29. Diagram of a Begg arch designed to achieve bodily movement of upper anterior teeth.

segments are not allowed to move forwards, so that anchorage must be supported extraorally or by means of intermaxillary traction. The 21/12 are now retracted with a removable appliance, whilst maintaining the incomplete overbite, and continuing to support the upper arch anchorage.

Fixed appliances will be required in those cases where it is necessary to correct axial inclinations, or rotations, or where the inclination of 21/12 need bodily retraction in order to achieve an aesthetically acceptable result.

Severe crowding. A greatly increased overjet is a characteristic feature, although this may be an indication of a marked dental base discrepancy. At the same time the impaction of teeth or their exclusion from the buccal segments is another feature of severe crowding. When this is combined with an increased overjet, the loss of four upper teeth will be necessary, together with expert space control in order to achieve sufficient overjet reduction to give an aesthetically acceptable result.

TREATMENT. The 7/7 should be extracted if 8/8 are present, but if absent the 7/7 should be retracted. When this has been accomplished the 6/6 are retracted one unit, supporting the upper arch anchorage with either intermaxillary or extraoral traction. In the next stage the 5/5 are retracted with an appliance which also incorporates a flat anterior bite plane to produce an incomplete overbite. Alternatively the 21/12 can be 'depressed' by a lower fixed multiband appliance if treatment is also being carried out in the mandibular arch.

The 4/4 should be extracted next, followed by retraction of 3/3, at the same time maintaining the incomplete overbite until finally the 21/12 can be retracted. Fixed appliances may be necessary if 21/12 require bodily retraction or rotation to produce a satisfactory alignment.

Class II Division 2 Incisor Relationship

The patient complains of protruding 2/2 or 3/3 often accompanied by irregular 21/12. Later in life there may be traumatic injury of the mucosa palatal to 1/1, and of the gingiva labial to 21/12 due to the increased overbite and reduced overjet characteristic of this malocclusion. Both the upper and lower labial segments are retroclined relative to their base planes.

Treatment

When the patient first attends during the mixed dentition phase the extraction of C/C will often allow 2/2 to drift distally and improve the appearance although not materially affecting the ultimate development of the malocclusion. However there is an increased likelihood in the upper buccal segments of excluding the $\overline{3/3}$ from the arch. As the premolars erupt they must be allowed to reach their full vertical development in order to achieve all possible reduction of the overbite, a fact which should be appreciated when considering the development of a dentition in this type of malocclusion. To accomplish this a removable appliance is used incorporating a flat anterior bite plane (see Fig. 7.19*b*). This can be designed to encourage a slight proclination of the upper and lower labial segments, which is also desirable, not only in order to improve the appearance but also reduce overbite and accommodate the teeth of the lower arch.

When the premolar teeth have erupted, the classical appearance is of $\underline{2/2}$ protruding, with the upper and lower labial segment retroclined to the base planes. The degree of crowding will determine what extractions are needed, and alignment of protruding $\underline{2/2}$ will require forward movement of their apices to ensure stability. This is best undertaken with fixed appliances. The object of lower arch treatment is to keep the lower labial segment as far forward as possible within soft tissue balance, in order to prevent further overbite increase which would arise following the collapse of the lower incisors.

Extraction of incisors, canines or $\overline{4/4}$ should be avoided. However, where teeth must be lost to relieve severe crowding, fixed appliances should be used not only to ensure controlled space closure but also to procline the $\overline{21/12}$ by as much as 5° into a position buttressing the upper incisors. This amount of proclination will compensate for any collapse which may have occurred as a result of early loss of deciduous molars or canines.

Severe crowding in the upper arch is uncommon because it is broad and U-shaped.

In mild crowding, extraction of $5/5$ will provide sufficient space to accommodate the excluded $\underline{2/2}$ or $\overline{3/3}$. Ocasionally the extraction of $\underline{7/7}$ may be preferred followed by distal movement of upper buccal segments, and retraction of $4/4$ and $\overline{3/3}$. If a removable appliance is used for this movement it should incorporate a flat anterior bite plane to help reduction of the overbite and carry clasps on $\overline{6/6}$ and $\underline{1/1}$. The appliance is designed to allow over-retraction of $\overline{2/2}$ by means of 0·7 mm buccal springs and at the same time the acrylic plate will require trimming to allow for the considerable palatal movement of the lateral incisors (Fig. 7.30) It is an advantage to move the apices of $\underline{2/2}$ labially and this can be achieved by applying pressure to the crown so that the cingulum impinges against the acrylic base of the appliance which acts as a fulcrum for this tipping movement. Occasionally it may be necessary to align the 1/1 with an appliance carrying a 0·7 mm bow.

Where there is a greater degree of crowding, extraction of 4/4 should be considered and a similar treatment instituted.

Those patients with Class II division 2 incisor relationship who have an increased overjet, will require treatment with fixed

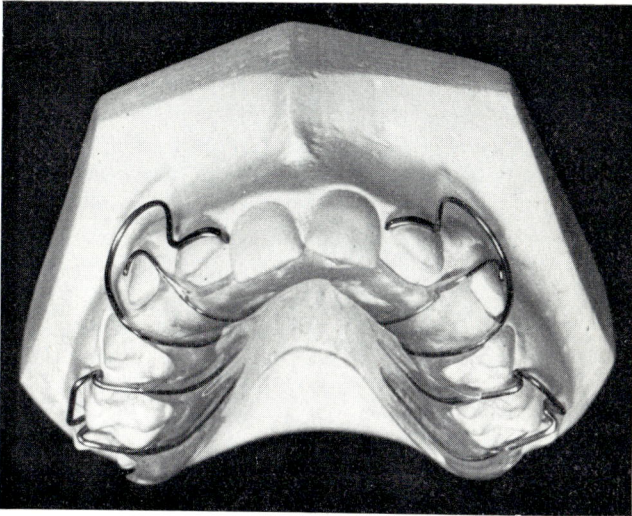

FIG. 7.30 Upper removable appliance to promote palatal movement of 2/2.

appliances if a Class I relationship is to be achieved since this involves uprighting the upper and lower labial segments by means of root-torque. In this way the reduction of the overjet can be accomplished at the same time as the control of space provided by extraction of premolar or molar teeth. Extraction of lower premolars allows alignment of lower incisors and will also permit Class II traction to be used, as anchorage support is required for the upper arch.

Class III Incisor Relationship

Treatment aims at eliminating crossbite in the anterior region, unilateral crossbite in the buccal segments if present, and also to relieve upper and lower arch crowding.

Factors influencing treatment

In patients of seven or eight years old, it is common to find one of the upper incisors occluding lingually to the lower incisors. On closer examination, it will be seen that during mandibular closure there is initial contact of these incisors with a lower tooth causing forward displacement of the mandible during further closure. This exaggerates the malocclusion and, in fact, there may be a Class I dental base, but due to this mandibular displacing activity, there is a Class III incisor relationship. Occasionally such patients may be shown to have a Class II division 1 incisor relationship and a Class II dental base relationship when in centric relation. The mandibular displacement should be eliminated at an early stage using a removable appliance (Fig. 7.31*a*, *b*).

Patients having a Class III incisor relation may have any of the three dental base relations, but more usually Class I or Class III, although rarely it may be Class II with a high maxillary-mandibular plane angle. They fall roughly into two groups depending on the size of the maxillary-mandibular plane angle: (*a*) the increased and (*b*) the decreased maxillary-mandibular plane angle groups. The significance of this is that the angle size affects the degree of overbite. The proclination of upper incisors using removable appliances will also result in a reduction of the overbite and this should be borne in mind when planning treatment, as these factors will affect the eventual stability of the occlusion.

Another feature of the malocclusion which should be remembered is that although maxillary growth may have almost ceased by twelve years of age, further forward growth of the mandible may continue until eighteen to twenty-one years and so contribute another 2-3 mm to the length of the mandible.

When the patients appear at a later stage of dental development, that is, when the premolars have erupted, more comprehensive treatment will be required to give a permanently stable result.

Treatment of the lower arch

It is unusual to find severe lower arch crowding in these cases, but when it does exist the $\overline{4/4}$ should be extracted provided that the remaining teeth are sound. Fixed appliances with bands on $\overline{7653/}$ $\overline{/3567}$ will then be necessary, not only for the retraction of $\overline{3/3}$ but also to maintain $\overline{53/35}$ in an upright position. If $\overline{3/3}$ are only tilted distally they will relapse and upright themselves when the appliance is withdrawn. When the retraction of $\overline{3/3}$ is complete, the $\overline{21/12}$

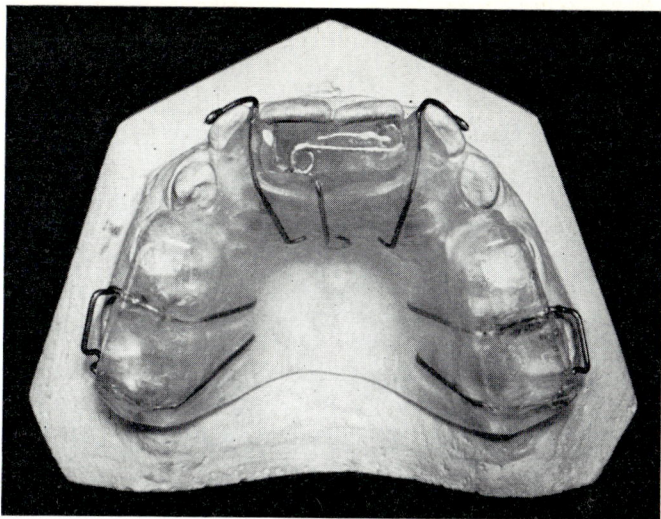

FIG. 7.31*a*. Upper removable appliance to procline 1/1.

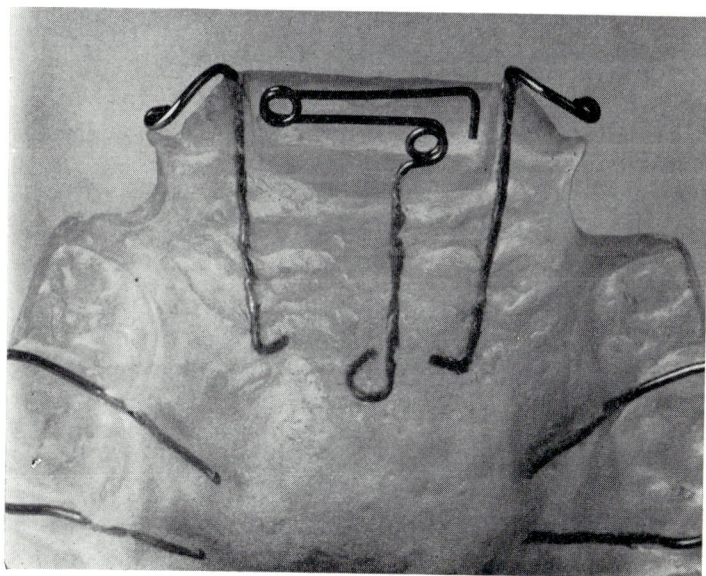

FIG. 7.31*b*. Detail of spring.

H

should be retroclined and aligned either by banding them or by use of Paul's tubing. Very occasionally it may be possible to retract the lower incisors bodily with a successful result, providing there is sufficient lingual bone.

The $\overline{6/6}$ may need to be extracted if they are very carious, but if this occurs the treatment will be lengthened considerably since $\overline{54/45}$ will have to be moved distally before the $\overline{3/3}$ can be retracted. Class III intermaxillary traction may be necessary to support the lower arch anchorage. Whether the space is already available in the lower arch or intentionally created by extractions to provide for a more favourable alignment of the lower labial segment, it is essential that in their new position they are in balance with the soft tissues, otherwise relapse is inevitable. Where the lower teeth are spaced prior to extraction it is doubtful whether the lower incisors can be retroclined, as the spacing suggests they are in soft tissue balance. Orthodontic treatment of these cases is to be avoided.

Treatment of the upper arch

Mild crowding is indicated where there is exclusion by one-third of a unit from the arch of $3/3$ or $5/5$ or slight imbrication of $21/12$.

Treatment in these cases should consist of extraction of $7/7$ and retraction of $654/456$ so that the $3/3$ can be accommodated within the arch and the labial segment aligned. As the buccal segments are retracted they undergo a slight expansion, but will require effective extraoral anchorage or alternatively Class II traction if lower space is to be closed (Fig. 7.32). Alternatively the $5/5$ may be extracted, the $4/4$ retracted and $21/12$ aligned with a removable or fixed appliance as indicated by the need to treat the axial inclination of the upper anterior teeth.

Average crowding indicated by exclusion of $3/3$ or $5/5$ combined with imbricated $21/12$.

In cases where there is average crowding, the $4/4$ should be extracted, followed by retraction of $3/3$, but before aligning the $21/12$ it is necessary to eliminate any initial contacts with opposing incisors. The decision to use either fixed or removable appliances depends upon the inclination of the teeth, but whatever spaces are left should be closed by Class III intermaxillary traction.

If the $3/3$ have a distal inclination their extraction should be considered, provided the $2/2$ and $4/4$ can make an acceptable contact so that the latter give a pleasant appearance when the patient smiles. On the other hand rotation of 4/4 will give a poor aesthetic result especially if these teeth have a pronounced lingual cusp.

Where the 2/2 are diminutive or poorly formed, a decision will be required as to whether they should be crowned or alternatively extracted so that the 3/3 may erupt as close as possible to the 1/1. If, however, spaces are already present in the upper arch the eruption of the 3/3 into the extracted 2/2 areas may produce a disappointing aesthetic result especially when the 3/3 crowns are small.

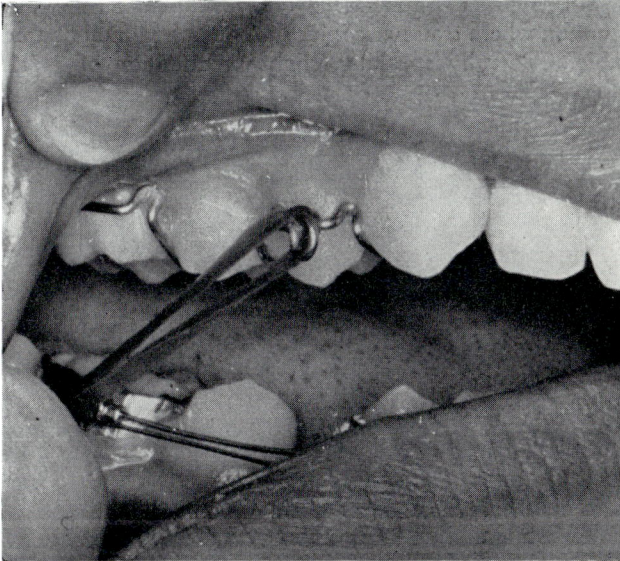

Fig. 7.32. Photograph of intermaxillary traction with elastics applied to an upper removable appliance.

Extraction of teeth in the upper arch should be accompanied by loss of appropriate lower premolars or molars in each instance.

Severe crowding will be indicated by the palatal exclusion of 5/5, buccal exclusion of 3/3, instanding 2/2 and perhaps some irregularity of 1/1.

Treatment should aim at relieving the crowding and producing an improved incisor relationship. Initially accommodation of 5/5 should be completed by use of an appliance to retract 6/6 after extraction of 7/7. Screws or springs may be the active component and anchorage should be supported extraorally or by the use of intermaxillary traction.

If the 6/6 have a poor prognosis their loss will allow alignment of 5/5. Following this, the second stage of treatment may proceed with the loss of 4/4 to allow accommodation of 3/3 and alignment of 21/12. Removable or fixed appliances should be used as indicated by the axial inclination of the teeth, and need for root movement. It is essential that the inclination of 21/12 relative to the maxillary plane should be determined accurately before treatment is undertaken. If the original position is one where 21/12 are already proclined, further proclination should be avoided since this will result in a situation where traumatic injury to the periodontal ligaments is inevitable. Generally speaking, slight proclination of 21/12 and retroclination of $\overline{21/12}$ is indicated in order to achieve a minimal overbite and overjet.

The aim in correcting the Class III incisal relationship is to buttress the upper anterior teeth against collapse and therefore upper arch extractions are to be avoided where possible.

Crossbite in buccal segments

A unilateral crossbite should be treated since it signifies that there is a mandibular displacing activity. It is corrected by using an appliance (Fig. 7.33) with a midline Coffin spring or screw aiming at bilateral expansion of the arch and molar blocks to disengage the occlusion. The treatment should aim at a slight over-expansion of the buccal segment, which should be retained for four months. Although the result will allow more space in the upper arch and sometimes eliminate the need for extraction, unfortunately it tends to decrease the overbite.

Bilateral crossbite is due to a narrow upper arch and since it does not cause a mandibular displacing activity, it should be accepted without any attempt at treatment.

Correction of rotated teeth

The problem of correcting rotated teeth is often a difficult one unless the treatment plan and appliance design are correct.

Rationale of treatment

1. Teeth are able to move mesially and distally provided there is free movement of the cusps in the fossae.
2. Space can be provided in the arch as in the case of lower

premolars which have rotated due to the early loss of a lower 1st molar.

3. Treatment of a rotated tooth is carried out prior to labial movement or retraction of incisors.

4. The treatment aims at over-rotating the tooth beyond its optimum position in order to allow for a slight relapse which nearly always occurs. It is retained in this position for nine months.

5. The aim of the treatment is to improve both the function and the aesthetics of the dentition.

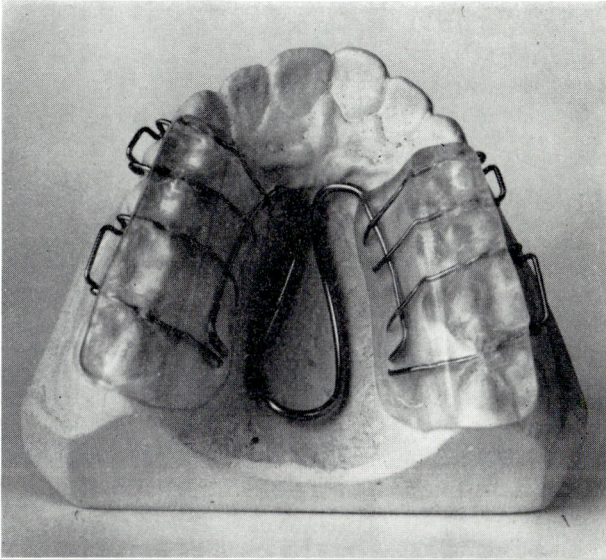

FIG. 7.33. Upper removable appliance with a Coffin spring to expand the upper arch and molar blocks to disengage the occlusion.

The teeth to be rotated are banded so that there is a definite point at which force can be applied. In the upper arch an incisor can be rotated by means of an upper removable appliance in conjunction with an auxillary spring (0·4 mm) wire attached to the banded incisor (Fig. 7.34). The spring is attached to the band by forming it into a 'pin' to fit into a box attachment welded to the band. The auxillary spring is about 15 mm long and at its other end is formed into a hook which engages the labial bow of the removable appliance. Since it is detachable the auxiliary can easily be replaced whenever necessary.

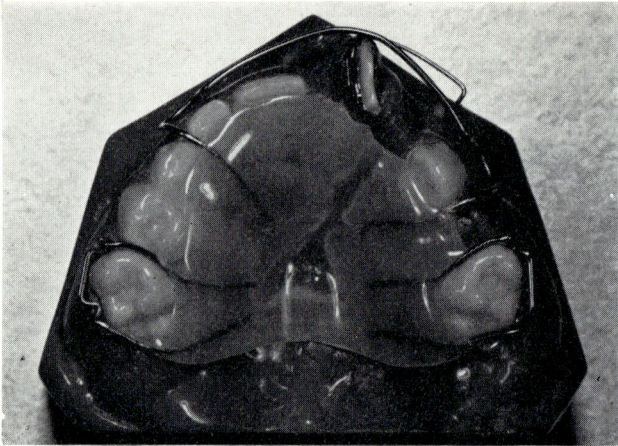

Fig. 7.34. Upper fixed/removable appliance to rotate /1.

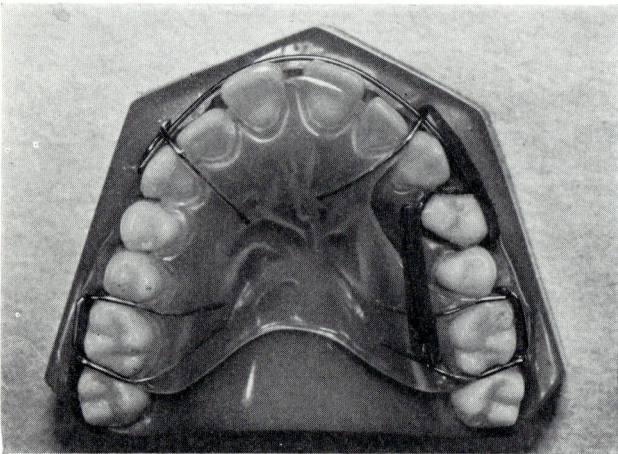

Fig. 7.35. Upper fixed/removable appliance to rotate /4.

For the rotation of premolars, a fixed-removable appliance is used (Fig. 7.35). Where the upper removable appliance is used to provide anchorage, the band on the /4 carries soldered, palatal and buccal hooks (double 0·5 mm soft stainless steel wire) which give definite points from which traction can be applied with latex bands. A mechanical couple is set up by which over-rotation of the tooth can be obtained.

A modification of the pin-and-tube appliance is shown for rotation of /2 (Fig. 7.36). The /246 are banded, 2/3 having been previously extracted. The round arch of 0·018 inch high-tensile wire can be activated to rotate and later retracts as it is adapted to fit the square section McKeag box. Ligaturing the sectional arch to the ripple bracket on /4 avoids arch distortion.

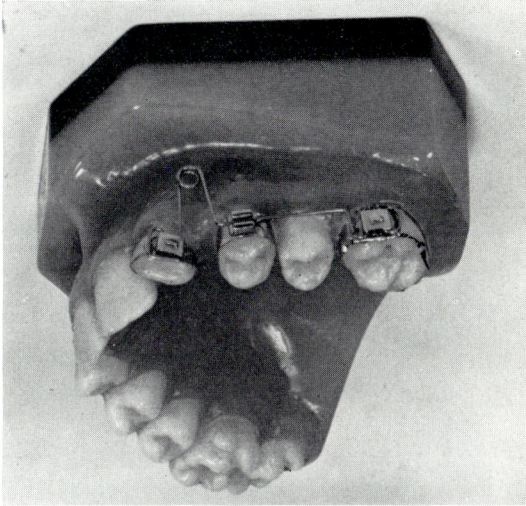

FIG. 7.36. Modification of loop and tube appliance to rotate /2.

A twin-wire arch appliance (Fig. 7.37) can be used for rotation of incisor teeth. As the degree of over-rotation cannot be obtained by tying in the twin arch to the brackets, even when offset, additions to the bands are made by using 2·5 × 0·25 mm soft stainless steel tape. The fulcrum for the rotation is therefore moved labially from the tooth surface. Grooves are either cut or moulded into the tape where the arch impinges to ensure that it does not slip from the fulcrum.

A Friel rotator is shown in a case where upper molar teeth have rotated forwards (Fig. 7.38). The tooth movements required were proclination of 21/12 and distal rotary movement of 6/6. Bands on 6/6 allow 0·35 mm auxiliary springs to be attached, so rotating them around the pivot provided by a 1·0 mm palatal arch seated in Vertical Selmer-Olsen tubes. As the palatal arch impinges on the anterior teeth, the slight forward reaction occurring during rotation of 6/6 will procline the upper incisors.

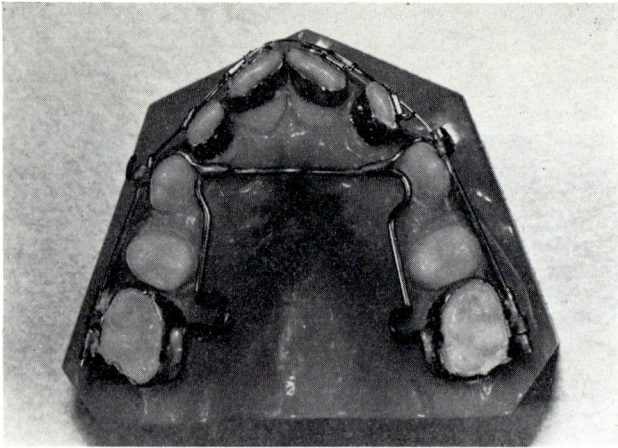

Fig. 7.37. Twin-wire arch appliance to rotate 21/12.

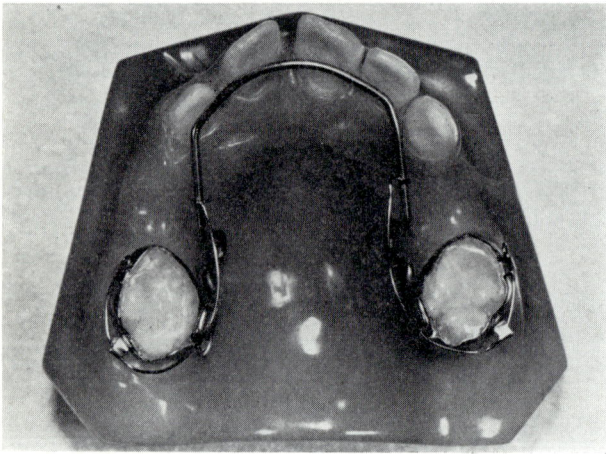

Fig. 7.38. A Friel rotation appliance applied to 6/6.

The rotation of teeth, using a multiband type of appliance can be carried out using:

1. Third power bends.
2. A modified Strang rotator.
3. Auxiliary arms from ripple brackets to the arch.

1. It is common to find lower canine teeth rotated, and prior to retraction or closing residual space in the arch, it is usual to align

them. This is carried out by using third power bends in a 0·016 inch high-tensile arch (Fig. 7.39). Such bends give added length to the arch, increasing resilience when it is required. If a plain arch is tied in it may be permanently deformed and produce no rotatory movement. The third power bends shown are partially tied to offset brackets, and on future visits more complete engagement of the arch in the bracket would produce over-rotation of the teeth concerned. Similarly, centrally placed brackets and eyelets may be used.

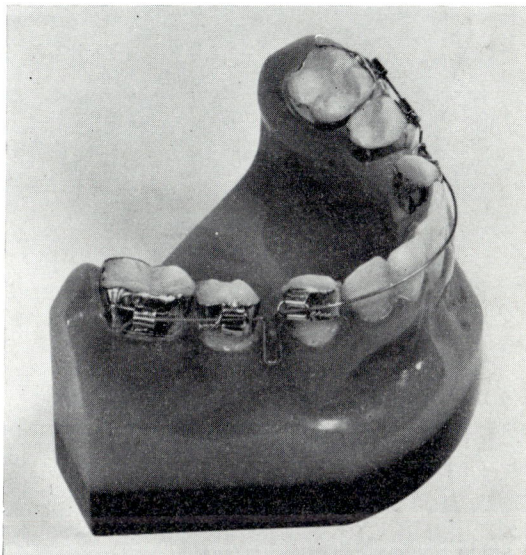

FIG. 7.39. Lower multiband appliance incorporating a third power bend to rotate $\overline{3}$/.

2. Rotation of molar and incisor teeth may be achieved by using a modified Strang rotator (Fig. 7.40). The premolar to be rotated has drifted as a consequence of early loss of the 1st permanent molar. The object is to move the distal aspect buccally and to do this an auxiliary of 0·016 inch high-tensile wire is attached to the buccal surface of the band. The auxiliary is formed and inserted into a tape tube on the disto-buccal area of the band. When the main arch is tied in, the loop on the auxiliary is tied to the arch to prevent unwanted movement of the tooth. The auxiliary being activated buccally, but its movement being prevented by the main arch, the distal aspect of the tooth is moved buccally and the mesial, lingually. The disadvantage of the method is the frailty of construction.

I

3. A variation of the method previously mentioned is where an auxiliary beam-type spring from a banded tooth, was attached to a removable appliance. Here the beam spring engages the main arch of a multiband appliance and in Fig. 7.41 the rotation of $\overline{5/5}$ is in progress.

The auxiliary spring of 0·016 inch high-tensile wire is threaded through the ripple channel on $\overline{5/5}$ bands, and a hook at its free end

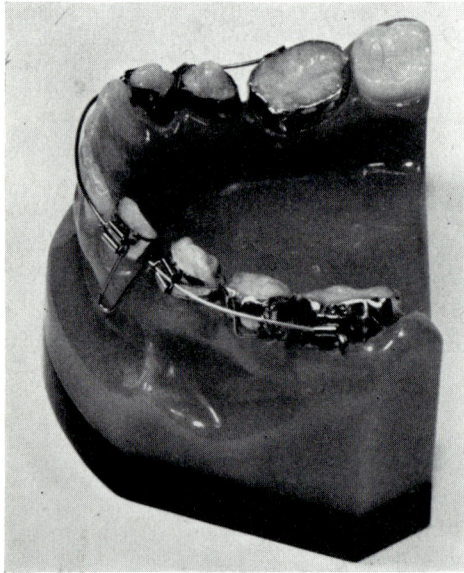

FIG. 7.40. Modified Strang appliance to rotate $\overline{/5}$.

engages the main arch. Such a method is useful for gross rotations where the deformation of a third power bend would be excessive. Over-rotation can be obtained by bending a step in the auxiliary arm.

The fact that there are numerous methods available for carrying out one basic type of tooth movement suggests that each tooth requiring rotation must be assessed on its merits, and no mechanical method should be used to the exclusion of all others.

Activation of Appliances
Removable appliances

Clasps and bows are adjusted, using universal- or spring-forming pliers so that the appliances stay firmly in the mouth during function.

Springs are adjusted so that the forces used to achieve tooth movement are within biological limits. A force of 25 g/cm² of root surface produces tooth movement and therefore as a guide 60-80 g force would be required to move cuspids and bicuspids. 30-50 g would produce movement of the upper incisors. These pressures may be measured by means of a Halda spring gauge, the arm of which is placed against the active spring and pressure applied until the

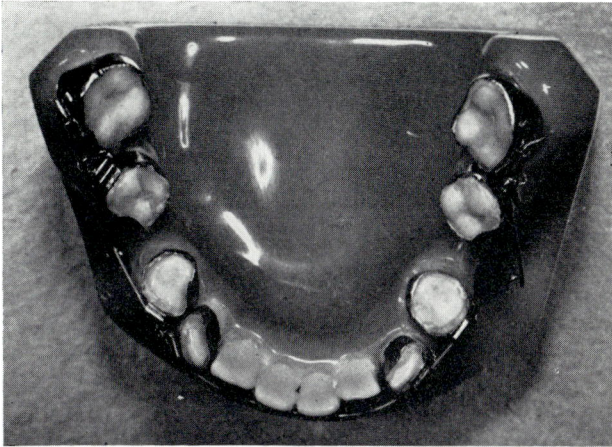

FIG. 7.41. Auxillary springs in association with a multiband
appliance to rotate $\overline{5/5}$.

spring is deflected to its initial position. In clinical practice, activation of a 0·5 mm hard stainless steel spring to one-quarter or one-third of the width of the cuspid or bicuspid provides the required force. Activating a 0·7 mm labial bow to twice the thickness of the incisal tips provided sufficient pressure to cause retraction of upper anterior teeth.

Screws are adjusted to stimulate tooth movement by opening the screw 0·2 mm, that is one-quarter turn at each visit. The opening of the screw must not exceed the combined widths of the periodontal ligament on either side of the tooth, which is approximately 0·4 mm, but screw adjustments should be made only once or twice per week. Under these conditions the teeth move at the rate of 1 mm per month.

Functional appliances move teeth under the stimulus of muscle activity combined with the special contouring of the base plate.

Fixed appliances

The high-tensile stainless steel wire used in multiband appliances is adapted by means of spring-forming pliers to produce forces on the teeth. These should be within the ranges already specified for individual teeth using removable appliances and although the force registered on deflection of the arch wire may appear greater it is, in fact, spread around many teeth, and it is acceptable for the individual teeth. Coil springs added to the wires should be used for mesiodistal tooth movement, ligating the coil from the tooth to be moved to the anchor teeth.

Elastic traction

Inter- or intramaxillary traction may be used with removable or fixed appliances, but due to the tendency for the traction to dislodge lower removable appliances, only a combination of lower fixed appliances and upper removable appliances is acceptable. The forces used may reach 150-180 g. Extraoral traction may be used in conjunction with removable or fixed appliances, and as the force is spread over many teeth, apparently great pressure may be provided. It has been our experience that providing the pressure does not keep the patient from sleeping, a biological force is being provided. The force measured at the attachment of the extraoral appliance may reach 400-500 g.

Maintainance of appliances

Removable appliances require to be worn whole-time by the patient. If they are not worn during the day or at night, they frequently become broken or lost. Economically the removable appliance is a costly item and if left out of the mouth it may be crushed underfoot or even thrown away by accident. There is also the temptation if other members of the family find the plate to 'test or adjust its springs' with a result that it may injure the tissues when re-inserted.

Occasionally the periphery of the base plate may be fractured and this may be repaired with cold-cure acrylic in the hydroflask or in some instances the appliance may be smoothed over and the breakage accepted for the duration of the life of the appliance. Breakage of the wire work frequently occurs near the point where the wire enters the base plate, but in this case replacement of the part is called for, since soldering is very difficult in this situation.

However, when the wire breaks at a point away from the base plate, such as at the arrow head of an Adam's clasp or on the corner of a labial bow, soldering of the broken part will provide satisfactory service for two or three months. It is important that the patient should inform the operator when appliances become damaged or a poor fit, or if unexpected dental pain occurs. For this reason an instruction sheet is supplied to the patient, and should include the following points:

1. It is most important that patients and parents cooperate in every possible way with the dental surgeon if the full benefit of orthodontic treatment is to be obtained.

2. Careful attention to cleanliness of the mouth and appliances is essential. If the appliance is removable, it should be cleaned with a toothbrush and paste after each meal to remove food debris. The teeth should be cleaned before the appliance is re-inserted. If a fixed appliance is in place, extreme care should be used when cleaning the teeth and appliance; the mouth MUST be kept scrupulously clean.

3. The appliance must be worn at all times, as only in this way will maximum benefit be obtained.

4. If for any reason the appliance cannot be worn (breakage or illness) the dentist should be informed immediately. A delay in this matter may lengthen treatment time considerably. Harm may result by waiting until the next appointment.

5. Adjustments should only be made by the dental surgeon except in the case of appliances incorporating screws, in which case they should be turned as prescribed in the direction of the arrow or towards the red dot.

6. Patients and parents are reminded that in the interests of dental health it is important to avoid eating sweets and biscuits between meals. Toffee should not be eaten at all.

7. It is essential that the patient attends appointments for routine dental care in addition to that required for orthodontic treatment. Failure to have fillings carried out may prevent a successful orthodontic result being obtained.

The operator must check the appliance thoroughly at each visit to see that the springs are applied correctly to the teeth and are not likely to fracture. It is important that he ensures the occlusion is not damaging the wire or the base plate and also checks that the appliance fits without rocking, since the latter indicates incorrect use and that it is liable to breakage. Where screws are being used, their length of travel should be determined by the operator when he sees the patient, to ensure that there is sufficient opening to carry the patient through to the next visit.

Care of fixed appliances

Fixed appliances frequently cause considerable tenderness of the teeth during the first week of wear and the patient should be reassured regarding this when they have the appliances fitted. There is also a certain degree of rubbing of the cheek against the appliance which causes white patches on the buccal mucosa, sometimes indentations, and very occasionally ulceration. The patient should report back if ulceration occurs, but as a temporary measure a small piece of soft wax can be applied to any rough areas of the fixed appliance to avoid undue distress. The patient should then report back to the surgery for adjustment and elimination of the rough areas. The use of Alastics (Unitek products: U.K. Agent—Orthomax, Bradford, England) has considerably reduced the complaints of this nature, particularly since ligature wires were easily dislodged during mastication and abraided the mucosa.

Breakage and deformation of arch wires occurs. This must be reported to the surgery so that the operator may correct the irregularities in the arch preferably by replacing it so that no unwanted tooth movements can occur. Bands may become dislodged and these should be replaced at once, and the patient instructed to report immediately they become loose, otherwise decalcification due to food lodgement will occur.

When fixed-appliance therapy is being carried out the anterior bands should be re-cemented at nine-monthly intervals and as far as the posterior teeth are concerned after twelve- to fifteen-monthly intervals to avoid the possibility of decalcification. Regular oral hygiene instruction is essential and should always be combined with a prophylaxis undertaken by the operator or his hygienist to avoid stagnation at the cervical margins of the teeth.

Extraoral appliances should be checked at each visit to ensure that they are not causing abrasion of the skin over the masseter area or rubbing the scalp and so causing patches of baldness, which may appear when these appliances have been incorrectly adjusted. For these reasons it is most important that the patients should be available to visit the surgery whenever necessary, especially when fixed appliances are being worn. Otherwise unwanted tooth movements will take place or relapses occur before the appliance can be corrected. The operator can help by giving regular appointments at four to six weekly intervals and spending adequate time at each visit to ensure that the appliances are well maintained.

Retention

When tooth movement is complete the teeth should be in a position of balance with the soft tissues, since only in this way will the occlusion remain stable. Record models should be made at this stage, since they are necessary in assessing any subsequent relapse. A retaining appliance usually of the removable type should be constructed, its purpose being to allow the periodontal tissues to re-establish themselves around the teeth whilst they are held in their new positions.

Design of retainer

The retaining appliance should be fixed in the mouth by means of clasps on the anchor teeth. The base-plate should be thin and well adapted around the necks of the teeth recently moved. A 0·7 mm stainless steel bow should be closely fitted to the labial surfaces of the teeth. Although there may be a temptation to convert the last active appliance into a retainer, this is seldom successful due to the design of the active components.

In cases where there is no adverse soft tissue pattern and no rotations, the retainer should be worn whole-time for three months and then three months at night only (from 6 p.m. to 8 a.m.). Where there is an adverse soft tissue pattern, retention is advisable for six months whole-time and three months nights only.

Management of teeth following rotation

Where a rotation has been corrected, the result should be retained for a period of nine months to allow complete reconstruction of the periodontal ligaments. In the majority of cases any rotations can usually be corrected during the first four months of treatment and subsequently retained whilst the remainder of the treatment is being completed. This effectively shortens the period which would have to be allowed purely for the retention of the rotated teeth.

When the retention period is completed, the appliance is withdrawn and the patient asked to return after three months for review. Thereafter annual and later biannual reviews are arranged until the age of eighteen years, so that the operator can ensure that the treated malocclusion remains stable into adult life.

8 Management of the Developing Occlusion

Effect of extraction of the deciduous teeth

Loss of deciduous incisor teeth will have little effect on the developing permanent dentition provided that potential crowding is minimal. Where crowding is present, mesial drift of $\overline{B/B}$ with loss of A/A, or of C/C with loss of $\overline{BA/AB}$, will occur and cause impaction of permanent teeth as they erupt. The treatment required is extraction of deciduous teeth to allow permanent teeth to erupt until the crowding is localised in the buccal segment, from whence permanent teeth can eventually be removed.

Unilateral loss of deciduous teeth may lead to movement of the centre line to the extraction side, and with this in mind, symmetrical loss is usually advisable.

Loss of deciduous canine teeth will allow spacing and alignment of permanent incisors, but at the same time, when crowding is present, the buccal segments tend to move forward and close the space, so excluding the permanent canines. Where deciduous canines have relatively high cusps, an initial contact may occur due to this, causing forward or lateral deviation of the mandible during closing. Loss of the canines or reduction of cusp height will serve to eliminate the displacing activity so that centric occlusion may again be achieved.

Loss of 1st deciduous molars has little effect on the majority of developing dentitions, except where crowding is extreme when the extraction space will close following tooth drift. In the child with strap-like lower lip the lower incisors will be able to retrocline in response to the soft tissue pattern.

Loss of deciduous 2nd molars is a more serious matter as the space available is usually taken up by the 1st permanent molar, which on moving mesially excludes the 2nd premolars. The upper 1st permanent molars usually rotate forward around the palatal root giving a contact with 1st premolars which is broad and less caries-resistant than normal. The lower molars tip mesially leaving a triangular space between molar and premolar which is prone to periodontal disease.

The loss of upper deciduous 2nd molars followed by forward

rotation of permanent molars and impaction of 2nd premolars leads to the need for lengthy orthodontic treatment where overjet reduction is eventually required. The extraction of 4/4 or 6/6 will only allow for 5/5 to be accommodated and where overjet reduction is also required, extraction of 7/7, retraction of 6/6, followed by eruption of 5/5 and loss of 4/4 will be needed. This may have been avoided had E/E been retained. It is well worth while spending time restoring deciduous molars in a case such as this.

Injuries to the primary dentition and the effects on permanent incisors

Traumatic injuries often lead to intrusion of BA/AB. The permanent incisors develop palatally and therefore, depending on the direction of intrusion, various disturbances of 21/12 may occur.

Frequently the deciduous teeth are displaced forward relative to permanent teeth and leave them undamaged. Should one of the deciduous incisors impinge on the permanent incisor crown when the crown is formed but the root is part formed, angulation of crown and root will result and the eventual eruption of permanent incisor prevented as described in Chapter 5. A firmness in the buccal sulcus may be the only indication of its presence. The dilaceration varies in degree but is usually in the apical third, and results in the failure of the permanent tooth to erupt, with consequent malocclusion caused by tooth-drift in the crowded mouth (Fig. 8.1). Deciduous incisors rarely suffer fracture of their crowns. Injury usually results in intrusion or dislocation or in more severe cases, loss of teeth and buccal plates of bone. Radical surgery in these cases may lead to distortion of the gingival margin in the permanent dentition and, for this reason, a conservative approach is recommended.

Submerged primary teeth

The 1st and 2nd decidous molars are most commonly affected— upper and lower. The teeth fail to develop with the surrounding alveolar bone and the condition is therefore one of lack of boney development rather than submergence (Fig. 8.2). The result is that the surrounding teeth continue to develop and the affected tooth is at a lower level. The gingival margin grows over it and in the long term the crown of the tooth may almost disappear, and the appearance may suggest that a tooth is erupting in the area. When submergence is complete, the space between crown and gingival margin

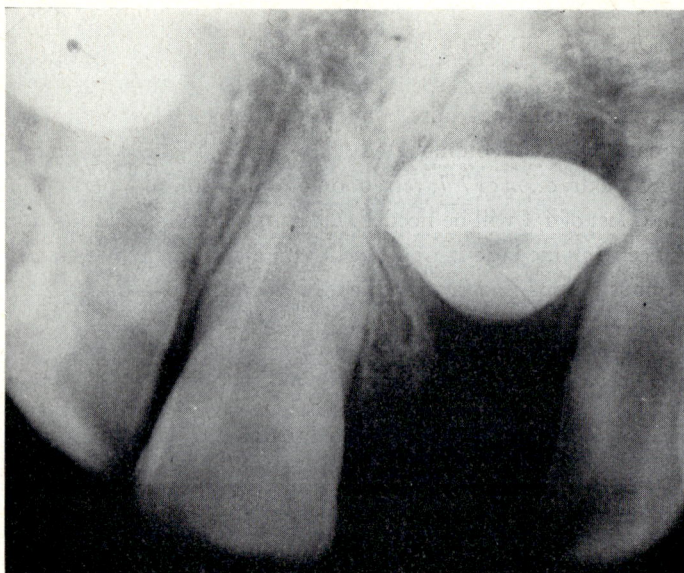

FIG. 8.1. Malocclusion caused by dilaceration of the central incisor in a crowded arch.

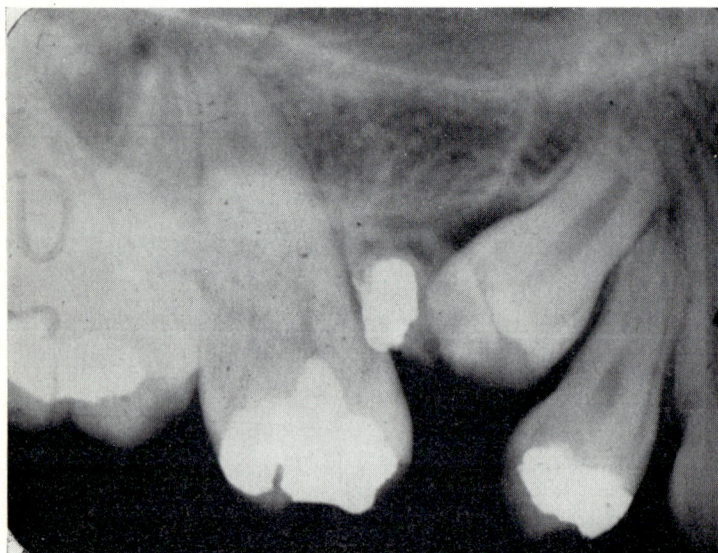

FIG. 8.2. Submerged upper 2nd deciduous molar, restored at an earlier stage, but now obstructing the normal eruption in the buccal segment.

may become infected. The adjacent teeth tilt and firmly wedge the submerged tooth. One serious consequence is that the premolar is prevented from erupting, and in all cases radiographs should be available to show the presence and position of the premolar teeth.

Treatment demands extraction of the submerging tooth at an early stage. Delay tends to make extraction more difficult due to the wedging effect of adjacent teeth. If the condition is allowed to remain undisturbed, the premolar may not be uncovered until its eruptive phase has passed and difficulty may be found in encouraging the permanent tooth to assume its occlusal level.

Loss of 1st permanent molars

The decision to extract the 1st permanent molar is often forced upon the dental surgeon, due to the high caries experience of some individuals. The outcome depends upon the dental age at which extraction of 1st permanent molars occurs, and the incisor relationship and degree of crowding of the teeth. The ideal case for loss of 1st permanent molars should present the following characteristics:

1. Class I dental base relation.
2. Class I incisor relationship.
3. Minimal crowding of the labial segments. If rotations are present they will not be corrected by this treatment and fixed appliances would be required.
4. Crowding in the buccal segments either present at this stage or potential as seen on radiographs.
5. A dental age of nine years, that is with 2nd molar crowns formed. The premolar teeth should be present in correct relation to the adjacent teeth.
6. The 1st molars should be carious as otherwise extraction of premolar teeth will certainly be preferable.

When 1st permanent molars are extracted in circumstances other than those described above, complications occur which increase the difficulty of orthodontic treatment. The path of eruption of the upper permanent molar in a crowded arch allows the 2nd premolar and 2nd molar to achieve an acceptable relationship. However, the lower 2nd molar has a more difficult eruption compared with the upper and frequently fails to close the space left by the extraction of the 1st molar. The 2nd molar crown frequently tips mesially due to drift (see Fig. 7.16) and also to occlusal pressures during its eruption, and it may also incline lingually. If the condition is then considered for orthodontic treatment, fixed appliances are required over an additional four-month period to upright the tipped lower 2nd molar following which space closure may be achieved in the usual manner.

In the cases of the extremely crowded upper arch when 6/6 are extracted prior to eruption of 75/57, the 2nd molars may then erupt and exclude the 2nd premolars from the arch. Should a Class II incisor relationship be present, reduction of overjet will not occur and there will be little improvement for accommodation of the upper canines. In this example loss of 1st molars will have done little to relieve crowding and have added to orthodontic treatment time to the extent of having to retract rotated 2nd molars prior to correcting the original malocclusion. A similar situation may occur in the very crowded lower arch.

A frequent occurrence in the lower arch is space between 1st and 2nd premolars following extraction of 1st molars. This occurs when the lower 2nd premolar originally had a distal inclination and loss of the 1st molar allows the premolar to erupt on this path, eventually preventing the mesial movement of the 2nd molar (see Fig. 7.17). In order to avoid this distal drift of the 2nd premolar, it should be allowed to erupt through the mucosa before extracting the 1st molar.

Generally speaking, in the upper arch the 2nd molar rotates mesially as it closes the 1st molar space, whereas in the lower arch the 2nd molar tips forward to leave a situation unacceptable from the periodontal and prosthetic standpoint, which, therefore, warrants orthodontic treatment (see Fig. 7.16). When 1st permanent molars are carious or heavily restored (two surface restoration at age eleven years) they may be the teeth selected for extraction in order to relieve crowding. However, even in optimal circumstances the utilisation of 1st molar space rather than 1st premolar space will add nine months to treatment time. It is therefore important to preserve 1st molars where possible as they are rarely the teeth of choice for extraction in order to correct a malocclusion.

Space maintainers

These are only infrequently required, as in the majority of cases crowding will eventually be present in the arch. Time and effort will be wasted maintaining space for individual teeth only to find that extractions are needed later and the remaining teeth require alignment with active appliances.

The use of space maintainers is therefore necessary when there is sufficient space for the teeth in the arch, but due to the eruption pattern, teeth which erupt at a later stage may be excluded from the arch. This situation arises commonly with 2nd premolars when 2nd deciduous molars are lost and the 1st permanent molars move one-quarter of a unit mesially. In a severely crowded upper arch the 1st molar may drift mesially to contact the 1st premolar.

Following loss of permanent incisor teeth, a space maintainer is indicated especially in the crowded arch, in order to prevent tooth drift into the space. It is a matter for consideration at the appropriate stage of development whether to align the remaining teeth, allowing that loss of one incisor will adequately relieve crowding, or to preserve space permanently with a partial denture or bridge, and relieve crowding by extraction in the buccal segments. Whatever is decided, controlled tooth movement, usually with fixed appliances, is indicated rather than uncontrolled tooth drift. When a space maintainer is indicated it should fit well around the adjacent teeth and preferably have clasps which engage these teeth, as in crowded arches the presence of erupting teeth may lead them to overlap the space maintainer. Acrylic teeth should be added to the space maintainer as required in order to provide the patient with a saisfactory appearance.

Space maintainers may be fixed or removable. The fixed type employ bands on the teeth adjacent to the space being preserved, with a 1 mm arch soldered between, avoiding the area where teeth are to erupt. The removable type clasps the teeth adjacent to the space being preserved, and the acrylic base is trimmed to allow eruption of teeth as this occurs.

Serial extraction

Serial extraction is designed for treatment without appliance therapy in the correction of malocclusion where there is crowding in the mixed dentition, and $\underline{21/12}$ have erupted in a Class I incisor relationship. It is advantageous to remove $\dfrac{C/C}{C/C}$ to allow $\dfrac{2/2}{2/2}$ to align. Later this is followed by removal of $\dfrac{D/D}{D/D}$ to allow $\dfrac{3/3}{3/3}$ to align, and the localised crowding in the $\dfrac{54/45}{54/45}$ area is then reduced by extraction of $\dfrac{E4/4E}{E4/4E}$ which will allow eruption of $\dfrac{5/5}{5/5}$. It is important that radiographs show before hand that all teeth are present and in correct developmental position, especially $\underline{3/3}$, and also that $\underline{4/4}$ are erupting ahead of $\underline{5/5}$, otherwise their removal will be difficult. If the axial inclination of $\underline{3/3}$ is unfavourable, fixed appliance therapy may be needed to upright them, and therefore serial extraction is not indicated.

The serial extraction technique localises crowding to buccal segments. It can be modified if one arch is crowded to allow relief in that arch only, while leaving the other to develop naturally. The system of serial extractions can also be adopted when there is crowding of the labial segments, with Class I incisor relationship associated with rotation of anterior teeth. These rotations can be corrected, using the appropriate appliance, as serial extractions proceed.

Digit sucking

Thumb sucking is a source of comfort to a child, who may resort to it when the domestic or school environment cause stress. Sometimes the cause of the discomfort is obvious, such as the competition with a new baby for the parent's attention. Under these circumstances the thumbsucking may be an attempt to resort to an earlier age-group and so recapture the parents' attention in that way. At a later age an unsightly appearance, such as caused by overweight, may lead to the need for comfort from digit sucking. In other cases it appears to be unrelated to environment or events and may start in the first few months of life and become an established habit which is particularly difficult to control if it persists into teenage.

The tongue, fingers and thumb may be involved. The sucking varies in intensity in different individuals, and when a firm grip is persistently taken on the digit a callous may form. The habit of placing the digit between the lips and teeth will produce an incomplete overbite or anterior open bite (see Fig. 2.38). This may be unilateral or bilateral. When the digit is not in place, the tongue moves forward to complete the anterior oral seal by contacting the lower lip. This is known as the tongue to lip resting posture.

The irregularity is seen in the deciduous dentition and produces a diastema between A/A. When the habit persists the anterior irregularity will be seen in the permanent dentition. In many patients the habit fades naturally during eruption of the permanent incisor teeth. However, when the habit continues it is advisable to persuade the patient to cease, and this is often achieved by leaving the parent in the waiting-room and discussing the matter directly and confidentially with the child. The dental surgeon should avoid embarrassing the child, since this results in loss of confidence.

A sympathetic talk with the older child will help to motivate him against such habits at school, although he is allowed to do it at home, but later, only in bed. As the young child falls asleep, the thumb or finger is removed from the mouth, so limiting the sucking time to less than one hour per day.

In some cases where the cooperation is poor, or the sucking drive is intense, removable or fixed appliances may be necessary in order to break the habit. The removable type should cover the hard palate and be divided with a midline split so that suction cannot be achieved, thereby reducing the satisfaction obtained from digit sucking (Fig. 8.3).

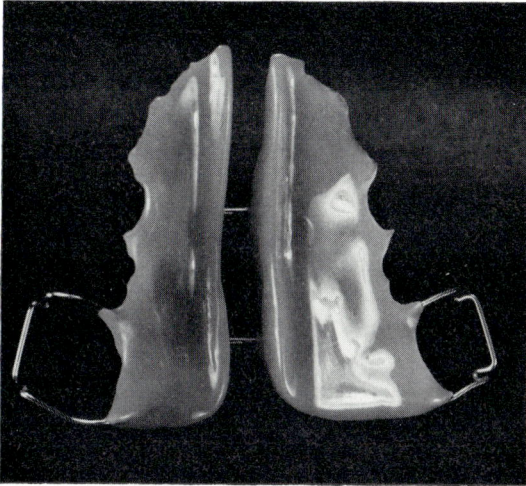

FIG. 8.3. 'Split-plate' worn to prevent persistent thumb sucking.

The fixed type, banding E/E or 6/6, has a palatal arch with rail guard welded anteriorly (Fig. 8.4). Since the appliance is fixed, care should be taken to ensure that the occlusion and the lower mucosa are unaffected during mastication. It effectively prevents the thumb from being sucked but ardent digit suckers, who are unable to control their desire to suck, may dislodge the appliance so that they can continue the habit.

Orthodontic treatment of non-vital teeth

Orthodontic tooth movement is dependent on healthy periodontal structures. The state of the pulpal tissue may also be affected by tooth movement. If the pulp is in a state of chronic or acute inflammation, tooth movement may lead to an exacerbation of the condition. Therefore, orthodontic treatment should be delayed in situations where the health of the pulp is in doubt following clinical and radiographic investigation, until the condition has been treated.

The orthodontic movement of teeth with satisfactory root fillings is carried out in the usual manner using fixed or removable appliances. A period of six months is allowed to elapse between the completion of endodontic treatment and tooth movement being recommenced.

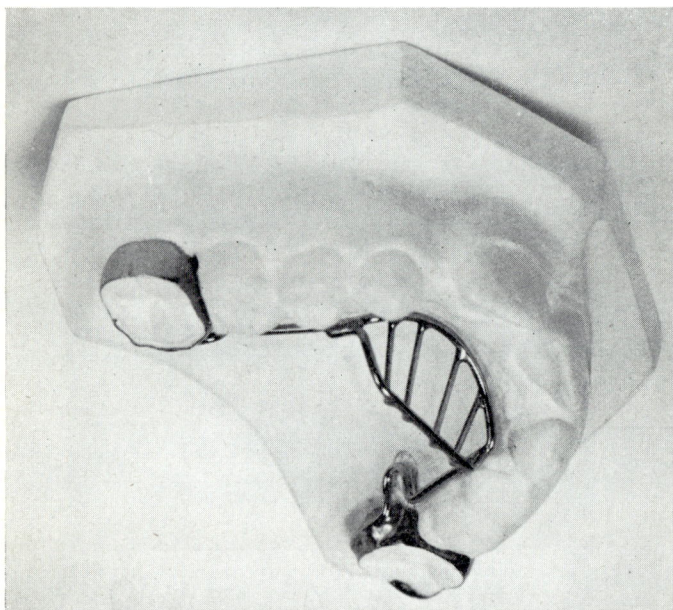

Fig. 8.4. Upper fixed appliance carrying a 'fence' to deter thumb sucking

Where apicectomy has been carried out, the fulcrum about which the tooth moves is altered in relation to the length of the root and there is more likelihood of crown tipping.

Occasionally, a tooth with a calcified pulp requires orthodontic treatment. This should proceed in the normal manner.

Speech therapy in relation to malocclusion

Speech therapy is the treatment of disorders of speech and language. The speech therapist and dental surgeon should work in conjunction with each other, the speech therapist treating the patient either before, or after, a course of orthodontic treatment. In cases where the malocclusion is untreatable and, as a result, speech is defective, the speech therapist helps the patient to compensate for the difficulty. However, it must be stressed that in other cases two children with the same dental abnormality may differ in their compensation for the disorder, because of factors such as intelligence, environment, parental stimulation and hearing.

Malocclusion affecting speech

1. **Developmental factors.** The development of articulation is a gradual process, the sounds of speech being acquired at different levels of maturation (Table 8.1).

TABLE 8.1

Age	Sounds acquired							
3	p	b	m					
4	t	d	n	k	g	ng	j	y
5	f	v						
6	th	s	z	sh	l			
7	r	wh						

The normal transition from deciduous dentition to permanent dentition may render speech defective for short periods, for example the loss of the upper deciduous incisors may affect *s*, which would then become *th*. The loss of teeth before speech patterns have become firmly established may make articulation difficult at a later stage. It is when these abnormal patterns become habitual and prolonged that speech therapy is indicated.

2. **Malocclusion.** *Malposition of individual teeth.* This may affect articulation, particularly of dental consonants, where speech involves the approximation of tongue and alveolus.

Adverse dental base relation. A prognathic or a retrognathic jaw relationship may make speech difficult and also uncomfortable to perform, and under these circumstances the speech is defective because the child speaks in whichever way causes least discomfort.

The establishment of an anterior open bite may produce poor articulation because of a defective oral seal and abnormal spacing at the front of the mouth.

SOUNDS AFFECTED BY MALOCCLUSION are shown in Table 8.2.

Over a lateral horizontal plane, speech may be rendered defective more specifically, for example when producing lateral consonants, particularly from affricates and sibilants. Examples are the *s* and *ch*, which are pronounced as the Welsh *Ll*.

TABLE 8.2

Class			Components		
plosives	*p*	*b*	*m*		
dentals	*t*	*d*	*l*	*n*	
fricatives	*f*	*v*	*s*	*z*	*th*
affricates	*sh*	*ch*			
semi vowels	*w*	*j*	*y*		

3. **Cleft lip and palate.** The speech therapist is a member of a team which treats children with cleft lip and palate and associated dental problems. With improved surgical techniques normal articulation usually develops spontaneously, and therapy mainly consists of assessment and advice, excepting where there are associated problems such as impaired hearing or reduced attendance at school.

Early surgery is an advantage to speech as consonants are developing in vocal play from the early months and in the case of cleft palate these activities will be abnormal.

Factors indicating the need for speech therapy include poor surgical result, residual faulty habits of articulation, tensions and effort, and the need for emotional support. The aim of treatment is to produce articulation accepted as 'normal', or where this is impossible, compensation and acceptance of limitations.

4. **Orthodontic appliances.** Orthodontic appliances rectifying malocclusion of teeth may render speech temporarily defective if the child does not adjust to the new shape of his mouth.

Speech therapy is not indicated unless faulty patterns remain after removal of the appliance.

5. **Stammering.** Stammering is a condition which is characterised by hesitations and/or cessations of sounds during the flow of speech. Factors which are thought to be responsible are still in dispute and are known to vary from individual to individual. There is, however, no evidence to suggest that a malocclusion *per se* may produce a stammer.

The majority of children pass through a period, around three years of age, when the speech lacks fluency and is unstable due to the immaturity of the articulatory patterns and of expressive linguistic ability. It is during this time that a malocclusion associated with other strongly influential factors may precipitate a stammer. Conversely, a child who is already stammering, and who has the added handicap of malocclusion, may associate difficulty in speaking with the disorder. The result of this may mean that the stammer is perpetuated through over-awareness of the orthodontic problem, but it is important to emphasise that a malocclusion is not likely in itself to give rise to this speech defect.

Additional Reading

Chapter 1

KILLEY, H. C. and KAY, L. W. (1969). *The Prevention of Complications in Dental Surgery*. Edinburgh and London: E. and S. Livingstone.

MCDERMOTT, J. F. (1963). Understanding the nature of children's reactions to dental experience. *J. Dent. Child.* **30**, 126.

TANNER, J. M. (1958). *Physical Maturing and Behaviour at Adolescence*. London National Children's Home.

Chapter 2

BALLARD, C. J. (1953). The significance of soft tissue morphology in diagnosis, prognosis and treatment planning. *Europ. orthodont. Soc. Trans.*, 143.

BAUME, L. J. (1950). Physiological tooth migration and its significance in the development of the occlusion. *J. dent. Res.* **29**, 123.

COOKE, B. E. D. (1958). Epithelial smears in the diagnosis of herpes simplex and herpes zoster affecting the oral mucosa. *Brit. dent. J.* **104**, 97.

DOWNS, W. B. (1952). The role of cephalometrics in orthodontic case analysis and diagnosis. *Am. J. Orthodont.* **38**, 162.

GREENE, J. C. and VERMILLION, J. R. (1964). The simplified oral hygiene index. *J. Amer. dent. Ass.* **68**, 7.

HARTLEY, D. T. (1956). The clinical assessment of the unerupted maxillary canine. *Dent. Practit. dent. Rec.* **6**, 279.

SARNAT, B. G. and SCHOUR, I. (1941, 1942). Enamel hypoplasia (chronological enamel aplasia). In relation to systematic disease. *J. Amer. dent. Ass.* **28**, 1989-2000 (1941); *J. Amer. dent. Ass.* **29**, 67-75 (1942).

THOMPSON, J. R. (1949). The rest position of the mandible and its application to analysis and correction of malocclusion. *Angle Orthodont.* **19**, 162.

TULLEY, W. J. (1954). Prognosis and treatment planning in orthodontics (Class II, div. 1). *Brit. dent. J.* **97**, 135.

Chapter 3

ANDREW, P. (1955). The treatment of infected pulps of deciduous teeth. *Brit. dent. J.* **98**, 122.

BENNETT, G. G. (1964). Disclosing solutions for pedodontics. *J. Dent. Child.* **31**, 131.

BUONOCORE, M. G. (1971). Caries prevention in pits and fissures sealed with an adhesive resin polymerised by ultra violet light. *J. Amer. dent. Ass.* **82**, 1090.

GUSTAFFSEN, B. E., QUENSEL, C. E., LANKE, L. S., LUNDQVIST, C., GRAHNEN, H., BONOW, B. E. and KRASSE, B. (1954). The Vipeholme dental caries study. *Acta odont. scand.* **11**, 232-364.

MASSLER, M., BERMAN, D. S. and JAMES, V. E. (1957). Pulp capping and pulp amputation. *Dent. Clin. N. Am.* 789-804, Nov.

WINTER, G. B., HAMILTON, M. C. and JAMES, P. M. (1966). The role of the comforter as an aetiological factor in rampant caries of the deciduous dentition. *Arch. Dis. Childn*, **41**, 207.

Chapter 4

DUDGEON, J. A. (1962). *Oral Pathology in the Child.* New York Int. Acad. of Oral Path.

TYLDESLEY, W. R. (1969). *Oral Diagnosis.* Oxford: Pergamon Press.

WALTON, J. G. and THOMPSON, J. W. (1970). *Pharmacology for the Dental Practitioner.* British Dental Association.

Chapter 5

ANDREASON, J. O. and HJORTING-HENSON, E. (1966). Replantation of teeth. *Acta odont. scand.* **24**, 263, 287.

COOKE, C. and ROWBOTHAM, T. C. (1960). Root canal therapy in non-vital teeth with open apices. *Brit. dent. J.* **108**, 147.

GLASS, R. L. and ZANDER, H. A. (1949). Pulp healing. *J. Dent. Res.* **28**, 97.

GROSSMAN, L. I. (1960). *Endodontic Practice.* Philadelphia: Lea and Febiger.

HALLETT, G. E. M. and PORTEOUS, J. R. (1963). Fractured incisors treated by vital pulpotomy: A report of 100 consecutive cases. *Brit. dent. J.* **115**, 279.

HOBSON, P. (1969). Pulp treatment of deciduous teeth. *Brit. dent. J.* **128**, 128.

LEWIS, T. E. (1959). Incidence of fractured anterior teeth as related to their protrusion. *Angle Orthodont.* **29**, 128.

MUMFORD, J. M. (1966). *Endodontics.* Oxford: Pergamon Press.

NYBORG, H. and SLACK, G. L. (1960). Clinical evaluation of pulpotomy. *Int. dent. J.* **10**, 452.

STEWART, D. J. (1964). Delayed pulpotomy in traumatised teeth. *Dent. Practit. dent. Rec.* **15**, 58.

Chapter 6

BOWLEY, A. N. and GARDNER, L. (1969). *The Young Handicapped Child*, 2nd Ed., pp. 134-164. Edinburgh: Livingstone.

EDELSTON, H. (1960). The anxious child. *Brit. dent. J.* **108**, 345.

PARNELL, A. G. (1964). Adrenal crisis and the dental surgeon. *Brit. dent. J.* **116**, 294.

RULE: D. C., WINTER, G. B., GOLDMAN, V. and BROOKS, R. C. (1967). Restorative treatment of children under general anaesthesia. *Brit. dent. J.* **123**, 480

STEWART, D. J. (1965). A dental service for children with bleeding disorders. *Brit. dent. J.* **119**, 544.

SWALLOW, J. N. (1964) Dental disease in children with Down's syndrome. *J. Ment. Defic. Res.* **8**, 102.

SWALLOW, J. N. (1969). The dental management of autistic children. *Brit. dent. J.* **126**, 128.

TOZER, R. A., BOUFLOWER, S. and GILLESPIE, W. A. (1966). Antibiotics for the prevention of bacterial endocarditis during dental treatment. *Lancet*, **1**, 686.

WEYMAN, JOAN (1971). *The Dental Care of Handicapped Children.* Edinburgh and London: Churchill Livingstone.

Chapter 7

ADAMS, C. P. (1964). *The Design and Construction of Removable Orthodontic Appliances*, 3rd Ed. Bristol: John Wright and Sons Ltd.

BALLARD, C. F. (1957). A Symposium of Class II div. 1 malocclusion. Morphology in relation to treatment planning. *Dent. Practit. dent. Rec.* **7**, 269.

GRABER, T. M. (1954). A cephalometric appraisal of the results of cervical gear therapy. *Amer. J. Orthodont.* **40**, 60.

PRINGLE, K. E. (1955). Long term results of orthodontic treatment. *Dent. Practit. dent. Rec.* **6,** 297.

TULLEY, W. J. (1959). The role of extractions in orthodontic treatment. *Brit. dent. J.* **107,** 199.

WILKINSON, A. A. (1948). The first permanent molar again. *Brit. dent. J.* **85,** 121.

Chapter 8

BRAITHWAITE, F. (1964). *Cleft Lip and Palate in Clinical Surgery*. Eds. Rob, C. and Smith, R. London: Butterworth.

KJELLGREN, B. (1947-48). Serial extractions as a corrective procedure in dental orthopaedic therapy. *Europ. orthodont. Soc. Trans.* 134-160.

LITTLEFIELD, W. H. (1952). Thumbsucking and its relationship to malocclusion in children. *Amer. J. Orthodont.* **38,** 293.

MORLEY, M. E. (1970). *Cleft Palate and Speech*. 7th Ed. Edinburgh: Livingstone.

SEIPEL, C. M. (1949). Prevention of malocclusion. *Dent. Practit. dent. Rec.* **69,** 224.

Index

Printed by T. AND A. CONSTABLE LTD.